Non-Emerging Adulthood

This book offers a therapeutic approach to a problem that many families and mental health institutions face: a growing number of adult-children who struggle to progress to a psychological, social adulthood. The family patterns that revolve around adult-children can remain inert for decades, are often resistant to conventional therapy, and can cause chronic suffering to adult-children, parents, and extended families. The authors present a guide that addresses parents of adult-children as suffering people in their own right and as essential to assisting their child into entering functional adulthood. The authors, one of whom is the originator of the Non-Violent Resistance Therapy approach (NVR), provide an intervention manual that implements NVR principles for helping families of adult-children. The book is based on the authors' ten-year journey of helping such families in cases where traditional interventions and therapeutic values seem not to work.

DAN DULBERGER is a marriage and family therapist, and a psychotherapist. He is internationally recognized as an expert in Non-Violent Resistance (NVR) therapy and as a developer of the approach's implementation for adult-children and their families. He teaches in the University of Calgary's Couple and Family Therapy professional certificates and diploma program.

HAIM OMER is a professor in the School of Psychological Sciences at Tel-Aviv University, Israel, and the developer of the Non-Violent Resistance (NVR) approach for parents, teachers, and other caregivers.

T0381694

Non-Emerging Adulthood

Helping Parents of Adult-Children with Entrenched Dependence

Dan Dulberger
University of Calgary

Haim Omer
Tel-Aviv University

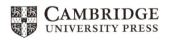

CAMBRIDGE
UNIVERSITY PRESS

University Printing House, Cambridge CB2 8BS, United Kingdom

One Liberty Plaza, 20th Floor, New York, NY 10006, USA

477 Williamstown Road, Port Melbourne, VIC 3207, Australia

314–321, 3rd Floor, Plot 3, Splendor Forum, Jasola District Centre, New Delhi – 110025, India

79 Anson Road, #06–04/06, Singapore 079906

Cambridge University Press is part of the University of Cambridge.

It furthers the University's mission by disseminating knowledge in the pursuit of education, learning, and research at the highest international levels of excellence.

www.cambridge.org
Information on this title: www.cambridge.org/9781108835688
DOI: 10.1017/9781108891240

First published 2021

A catalogue record for this publication is available from the British Library.

Library of Congress Cataloging-in-Publication Data
Names: Dulberger, Dan, author. | Omer, Haim, 1949– author.
Title: Non-emerging adulthood : helping parents of adult children with entrenched dependence / Dan Dulberger, Center for Nonviolent Resistance, Haim Omer.
Description: 1 Edition. | New York : Cambridge University Press, 2021. | Includes bibliographical references and index.
Identifiers: LCCN 2020049455 (print) | LCCN 2020049456 (ebook) | ISBN 9781108835688 (hardback) | ISBN 9781108891240 (ebook)
Subjects: LCSH: Parent and adult child. | Adult children – Family relationships. | Adulthood.
Classification: LCC HQ755.86 .D85 2021 (print) | LCC HQ755.86 (ebook) | DDC 306.874–dc23
LC record available at https://lccn.loc.gov/2020049455
LC ebook record available at https://lccn.loc.gov/2020049456

ISBN 978-1-108-83568-8 Hardback
ISBN 978-1-108-81302-0 Paperback

Contents

Introduction   *page* 1

Why NVR?   2

AED, the Intervention and Global Diversity   9

A Word of Caution   10

With Gratitude and Acknowledgment   10

1   The Adult-Child: Functional and Dysfunctional Dependence   11

The Age of Emerging Adulthood   14

From Crisis to Failure: the Role of Parental Uncertainty   15

A Realistic Goal: Functional Dependence   17

Identifying Dysfunctional Dependence   18

Entrenched Dependence from Childhood to Adulthood   32

2   NVR and Accommodation   34

The Adult-Child Refuses Therapy   35

The Adult-Child Agrees to Therapy, but AED Persists   35

Parents Are Advised to Show Unconditional Acceptance   35

Parents Are Advised to Be Tough   36

The Decision to Work with the Parents without the Adult-Child's

   Involvement in Therapy   36

The Narrative of Total Responsibility: Past, Present and Future   38

The Effects of Parental Accommodation   39

Parents' Difficulties in Stopping Accommodation   40

Dealing with Parental Objections   41

Treatment Goals   46

3   The Intervention   47

Settings and Course   47

The Opening Stage   49

The Announcement   57

Support   61

The Supportive Role of Other Professionals   67

The Process of De-Accommodation   69

The Conclusion Stage   78

4 Suicide Threats   81
   The NVR Program for Suicide Threats   83
   A Detailed Case of Suicide Crisis   90
   Indications and Contra-Indications for Using NVR in Situations
      of Suicide Threat   93

5 Helping Parents of Children and Adolescents at Risk of Failure
   to Emerge   95
   Digital Abuse   96
   School Refusal and Social Withdrawal   101
   Children with "Tyrannical Behaviors"   103
   Irresponsible Financial Behavior   105

6 Addressing Entrenched Dependence in Special Contexts   109
   Emergencies   109
   Worrisome Conditions   111
   Aged Parents   113
   NVR in Psychiatric Contexts   114
   NVR in the Psychiatric Ward   115

7 Survival Mode: the Adult-Child's Experience (by Ohad Nahum)   123
   Meeting the Adult-Child   123
   Developmental Factors of the Adult-Child's Experience   124
   The Adult-Child Experience   127
   The Therapeutic Encounter with the Adult-Child   131

   Conclusion   139

Bibliography   142
Index   147

Introduction

This book is a guide for therapists working with families of adult-children who are dependent on their parents in highly dysfunctional ways. It is based on 10 years of our clinical work with hundreds of such families. It summarizes what we have learned about the use of Non-Violent Resistance (NVR) therapy in such cases, and shares what we learned about the processes of *entrenched dependence*, *accommodation* and *de-accommodation* and their roles in perpetuating or alleviating these families' sufferings.

Since 2009, we have been using the concept of *Adult Entrenched Dependence*[1] (AED) to refer to an interpersonal pattern that forms in certain families between young adults or adolescents and their parents. Most of these adult-children live in the parental home and are usually not in employment, education or training. At the core of AED lies the perception – shared by the adult-child and the parents – that the child is inadequate and incompetent. This perception leads the parents to feel obliged to protect and shelter the adult-child. The adult-child, in turn, feels they cannot live without the parents' services. Whenever parents try to break out of their role, the adult-child reacts harshly. Over time, both sides come to experience this condition as inescapable. AED can persist in families for decades.

Research into adult childhood is still in its infancy (Pozza et al., 2019), but there are many indicators that this is a wide and growing social phenomenon. It is estimated that a total of 40 million adolescents and young adults in Organisation for Economic Co-operation and Development (OECD) countries are not in education, employment or training (NEET), and almost two thirds of that population (28 million young people across the OECD) are not even looking for work (OECD, 2016; 2019). Psychiatrists and psychotherapists are increasingly concerned about adolescents and young adults who are socially withdrawn and live secluded in their home or their room (Li & Wong, 2015; Pozza et al., 2019; Uchida & Norasakkunkit, 2015). Studies of adolescents at high suicide risk have identified a large category of youngsters described as

---

[1] Originally we termed the condition "entitled dependence." We now prefer the term "entrenched dependence" because it is less judgmental.

being "at silent risk for psychopathology and suicidal behavior," who are characterized by a sedentary lifestyle, decreased sleep and high media usage (Carli et al., 2014). In our experience, most cases of AED fall into those categories. The fact that adult-children are often introverted and socially avoidant does not prevent many of them from voicing their demands in highly vocal, if not downright violent, ways. Although adult-children are mostly homebound, many of them show financial and social irresponsibility, as well as addictive behaviors.

At the very center of our understanding and treatment of AED lies the process of accommodation. Parents accommodate to their child's demands and expectations, when they persistently adapt their attitude, behavior and rules to prevent their child from suffering. Accommodation can be voluntary, when parents act out of compassion for their child, or forced, when they feel coerced into accommodating by the child's extreme reactions. Accommodation has been shown to perpetuate anxiety, avoidance and dysfunction in children and adults with a variety of disorders (Shimshoni et al., 2019). Parental accommodation also predicts failure of individual treatment for the child (Garcia et al., 2010).

Why NVR?

Our intervention for families with AED is based on the NVR approach. NVR is an approach to families, schools and communities that is inspired by the doctrine championed by Mahatma Gandhi and Martin Luther King. At first view, it may seem puzzling that an approach that was developed for resisting political oppression effectively and morally should be found relevant for helping parents of children with behavior problems, at any age. Parents are not usually in a position of weakness relative to their children, nor do they experience themselves as oppressed. Nevertheless, the moment we understood that the principles and methods of sociopolitical NVR could help in our therapeutic work with parents, enormous possibilities were opened. To understand this, we must recapitulate what, in our view, was missing (and still is) in psychotherapists' work with parents.

Many parents who come for help are confronted with highly stressful situations that require their response: a boy beats up his sister and humiliates her before her friends; a teen shuts himself up in his room after voicing dire threats; or the parents receive a call from the police that their daughter has been found totally drunk. These and other acute situations require a parental reaction. And the parents do react, for remaining helpless and in extreme worry is also a reaction, though probably not a very helpful one. Very often parents come for therapy with such a sense of urgency.

In such situations, the parents often feel they need a practical and simple solution, a clear sense of direction. The reason they need it to be simple is that they are so stressed and confused that they cannot process very complex information. But we, psychotherapists, are not at our best with simple solutions. We are trained to search for complexity. We tend to be suspicious of simple explanations. Maybe this is one of the reasons that attracts us to the profession: the wish to search for what is not obvious, to trace richer and hidden processes. This disparity between the parents' immediate need and the counselor's tendency to focus on complexity may be a bad sign for the burgeoning therapeutic alliance.

This was the first challenge that we faced in developing an approach for helping parents of impulsive, violent or self-destructive children. We had to find a way to give the parents from the very outset a clear sense of direction, a kind of "parental-North" by which they could orient themselves. Something they could identify with, which would reduce their confusion and helplessness and make them feel they had a therapeutic partner who was mindful of their distress and sense of urgency. We wanted an initial guiding concept that would make the parents come out of the first encounter engaged and hopeful.

The concept of *parental presence* seemed to fulfil this role in a promising way. When helpless and worried parents came to us, we found that talking to them about increasing their presence in the life of the child and the family had an immediate engaging effect. We defined parental presence as the experience inherent in acts that convey the message, "I'm your parent. You can't fire me, divorce me or paralyze me. I'm here and I'll stay here." When we talked to parents in this vein, they became alert, responsive and motivated. The concept of parental presence seemed to galvanize them into a readiness to listen and act that was all but lacking in their previously defeated stance.

In the initial years of our work with parents, parental presence remained our major concept. We searched for ways in which parents could manifest their presence, how they could regain their voice, their place and their influence. We profited greatly from the work of Gerald Patterson, Salvador Minuchin, Jay Haley and Milton Erickson. But we always tried to subsume our borrowings from these various masters under the concept of parental presence. In this way, our work and message remained unified, although we borrowed eclectically from many sources. We gradually came to emphasize that not only the child should experience the parents as present, but also the parents themselves should feel that they had a voice, filled space, had weight and significance in the life of the family. This work culminated in the publication of *Parental presence: Reclaiming a leadership role in bringing up our children* (Omer, 1999).

When I (Haim Omer) was writing that book, I became aware of cases in which the idea of parental presence was misinterpreted. Some parents understood it as meaning they should achieve full control over the child. This interpretation might lead some parents to go home and set up barricades, conveying inappropriately dominant messages. Thus understood, parental presence could lead to escalation. Those difficult cases led me to add a chapter to the book, proposing possible ways to reduce the escalation that might arise as a consequence of the parents' manifestation of decided presence. With the addition of this chapter, I was able to publish the book without worrying too much about the potential negative consequences of its message.

But this ad hoc solution was insufficient. The danger of escalation is not just a casual consequence of the parents' manifestation of presence but is intrinsically connected to it. It is almost the other side of the coin. Many parents lose their presence precisely because their attempts to manifest presence lead to sharp reactions by the child and to frightening escalation bouts. Considering escalation as a possible side effect that could be remedied by palliative measures would not do. Presence and escalation had to be considered in their intrinsic mutual connection. NVR provided an answer to this challenge.

NVR is probably the only model of social struggle that is carried out by and through the personal, emotional and moral presence of the activists. The fight is not conducted by throwing stones, arrows, spears and bullets from a distance, but by the determined presence of the activists, which conveys the message "We are here. We stay here. We won't budge." NVR is also the only kind of resistance in which the activists are rigorously trained to avoid all acts of violence, as well as all provocations, denigrations and offensive acts that might lead to escalation. The reason is both moral and strategic. The force of NVR is a function of its ability to stimulate positive voices in the adversary camp, voices that are opposed to the continuation of their own violent and oppressive acts. These positive voices say: "They are the moral side. We are the bad guys." These voices, however, can only be efficiently fostered if the resisting camp avoids violence and deliberate offensive acts, which would justify the dominant side in pursuing its oppression.

Sociopolitical NVR did far more to further our approach to parenting than showing that presence and escalation are two sides of the same coin. The reason is that leaders like Mahatma Gandhi and Martin Luther King were not only inspiring political figures but also master strategists. They created a detailed lore about how to translate those principles into day-to-day practice. They developed cadres of trainers and field leaders that helped transform a moral political philosophy into a highly effective resistance machine. Fortunately, the richness of NVR's principles, strategies and tactics found their ideal historian and codifier in the figure of Gene Sharp. His classic book, The politics of nonviolent action (1973), is like a Talmud of NVR, providing guidelines for every imaginable situation and detailing each tool of resistance in all contexts of implementation.

Thus, the work of translating sociopolitical NVR into the family context was rendered possible. With the help of a few dedicated students, each intervention, strategic principle, tactical measure and training idea was examined in detail for its potential to the field of parenting. The combination of this work and our previous experience with parental presence led to the founding work of NVR (Omer, 2004b) and, more recently, a new edition: *Non-violent resistance: A new approach for violent and self-destructive children* (Omer, in press). Each and every principle, strategy and practical step in that book combines decided parental presence with the prevention of escalation. The book, and its treatment manual in the third chapter, became the basis of our treatment program and gave us a good starting point for our research program.

The next step that made NVR clearly relevant for cases of AED was the demonstration that adaptations of the NVR model for violent and self-destructive children were also effective for children with anxiety and other internalizing disorders. The first systematic adaptation of NVR to children with an internalizing rather than externalizing disorder was the Supportive Parenting for Anxious Childhood Emotions (SPACE) Program. The ration-ale for applying an NVR-based approach to those families was due to the parents' loss of their personal space (hence the acronym) on account of their child's anxiety disorder (Lebowitz & Omer, 2013). The loss of the parents' space is illustrated by the fact that many of them lose their ability to have a room that is really their own, to control their own time, to meet with friends, to go out as a couple or manage the house as they see fit, because of the requirements posed by the child's anxiety. These situations are also typical AED. A set of practical tools is included in SPACE to help parents identify the various forms of accommodation they provide, implement detailed plans for reducing accommodation and strategies for coping with the child's harsh responses. It is a quintessential model for how NVR can be translated for a condition with very different requirements than those of externalizing problems for which the approach was first formulated. In addition, SPACE and other adaptations of NVR for internalizing disorders showed themselves effective for children with various anxiety disorders, obsessive-compulsive disorder (OCD) (Lebowitz & Omer, 2013) and High Functioning Autistic Spectrum Disorder (HFASD) (Golan et al., 2018). It was not only as effective as Cognitive Behavioral Therapy (CBT) for the child (Lebowitz et al., 2020) but showed similar results with children who refused to accept treatment, thus making CBT not applicable (Lebowitz et al., 2014). Non-Violent Resistance (Omer, 2004a; 2004b, in press)[2] is well suited to help parents reduce accommodation and break out of the oppressive dysfunctional bond that keeps them and the adult-child chained to each other. The reasons are manifold:

---

[2] See www.haimomer-nvr.com/ for a fuller reference list of NVR-related publications.

(a) NVR sensitizes parents to situations where they are exploited and oppressed. In this respect NVR for parents follows in the footsteps of its sociopolitical model. The first step of NVR as a form of political struggle is to create awareness that the victims' submission is not preordained by God or nature. Similarly, the first step of parental NVR is to enhance the parents' awareness that their feeling of being obliged to service their adult-child is not a necessary consequence of the child's condition, but is often a result of habit, anxiety and coercion. When parents understand the destructive effects of accommodation on the adult-child, they are quick to perceive the damage it also inflicts on their life and on that of their other children.

(b) It helps parents to protect themselves, regain their agency and reclaim their personal space.

(c) It reduces the danger of escalation (Lavi-Levavi et al., 2013), which is usually what keeps parents in total fear of undertaking the necessary changes.

(d) It redeems parents and the family from isolation (van Holen, 2016; 2018). As will be seen, isolation is one of the important factors perpetuating AED. The passage from loneliness to support is key to empowering parents to liberate themselves and their child from their mutual trap.

On the conceptual side, this book offers a model for understanding the dependence bond that develops between parents and child in AED. When we first met families of adult-children, the literature describing the kind of family interactions we were witnessing was scarce. There were some references in the classical family therapy literature (e.g., Haley, 1980), mostly to a specific diagnosis, such as schizophrenia. Gradually, articles inspired by Dialectical Behavior Therapy (e.g., Ben-Porath, 2010; Zalewski et al., 2018) appeared, describing the mutual problems in emotional regulation between parents and very unstable young adults, as well as attempts to improve the child's condition by better parental emotional regulation. There is of course a lot of literature on various psychopathological conditions of young adults but very little on the special kind of dependence bond that we witnessed again and again. We therefore experienced AED as an uncharted territory and gained knowledge of it mainly by our own clinical observation. We now believe that the dependence bond typical of AED may not only be an important factor in mental health but also a growing social phenomenon deserving wide interdisciplinary research.

On the therapy side, this book offers a manual of NVR for AED. It is based on years of practice and refinement over hundreds of cases and is the latest in a series of manualized implementations of NVR for a variety of conditions, such as: conduct and oppositional-defiant disorders (Omer, 2004b), Attention Deficit Hyperactivity Disorder(ADHD) (Schorr-Sapir, 2018), anxiety disorders (Lebowitz & Omer, 2013), youth delinquency (Lothringer-Sagi, 2020), unbalanced diabetes (Rothmann-Kabir, 2018), computer abuse (Sela, 2019), dangerous teen driving (Shimshoni et al., 2015) and avoidant/restrictive food eating disorder (Shimshoni & Lebowitz, 2020). Additional NVR manuals were developed not on the basis of diagnosis but in contexts of implementation, such as foster parents (Van Holen et al., 2016) and psychiatric wards (Goddard et al., 2009).

To date, one clinical study of 27 families that have undergone our intervention has been published (Lebowitz et al., 2012). Since then, we believe our approach to have become ripe for further research and hope that this book will inspire an expansion of its evidence base.

We noted earlier in this section that little scholarly work on families of adult-children was available to support our earlier clinical explorations. What we did find in abundance, however, was a supply of slang and derogatory terms to denote the adult-children we were studying. Terms like "entrenched dependence" and "adult-children" might perhaps be understood as adding to this stigmatic vogue. That is categorically not our intention. To us, entrenched dependence does not reflect any "bad attitude" or "negative motivation," but a systemic pattern that involves both the parents and the child. We do not view AED as a psychopathological entity residing within the adult-child's mind. On the contrary, we view it as subsisting because of the special kind of dependence bond that develops between parents and child. Our work strives to transform this systemic pattern. The fact that this effort can be successful illustrates how context-dependent AED is.

Similar considerations apply to our use of the term "adult-child." The paradoxical connotation here is intentional, as it reflects a social reality. Coming of age has never been more difficult than in our era of *extended* adolescence and *emerging* adulthood. Considering this difficulty, failures of emergence are to be expected, leaving millions of persons and their families outside normative discourses on childhood, adolescence and adulthood. The figures we quoted at the beginning of this chapter about the incidence of NEET persons in OECD countries speak for themselves. Stigmatizing or pathologizing these people is a way of disowning social responsibility for their condition.

This book comprises the following chapters: Chapter 1 (The Adult-Child: Functional and Dysfunctional Dependence) links AED to the labyrinth of emerging adulthood (Arnett, 2004), describing it as a failure to emerge. A child's dependence on parents can be characterized as functional or dysfunctional. We present ways to differentiate between the two. We clarify that the goal of our approach is not to pursue a mirage of "independence" (which we view as a rather problematic goal) but helping transform dysfunctional into functional dependence. The main changes we try to promote are: (a) developing a time perspective that allows parents to strive for better functioning; (b) helping parents to move from personal effacement into presence; (c) releasing parents from their "sacrifice mentality"; (d) helping parents through a process of de-accommodation; and (e) identifying and resisting various forms of violence, blackmail and exploitation.

Chapter 2 (NVR and Accommodation) describes why parental NVR is well suited to treating AED. We describe why attempts at individual therapy for the adult-child or traditional parental counseling may fail. These failures have different forms, such as: (a) the adult-child refuses therapy; (b) the adult-child accepts therapy, but AED persists; (c) the parents are advised to show unconditional acceptance, but the dependence bond remains unaffected; or (d) the parents are advised to be tough but are daunted when they stumble on frightening escalation. We argue that parents are almost invariably the motivated partners, that they deserve to be viewed as clients in their own right, and that involving the adult-child would distract the parents and the therapist from their job. The chapter concludes with a description of treatment goals and of what changes can be realistically expected.

Chapter 3 (The Intervention) presents a detailed presentation of the NVR manual for AED. The intervention is not described session per session, as this would hinder adaptation to the special characteristics of each family. The manual specifies the essential treatment stages, the goals and tasks involved at each stage, and ways of dealing with typical parental concerns. This type of manual has been shown by previous research on NVR to guarantee satisfactory uniformity, as well as serving as a basis for the performance of treatment integrity checks (a central element in research). The treatment's *opening stage* is devoted to: building the therapeutic alliance, reframing the problem in ways that allow for new options, discussing parental accommodation, working on the parents' assumption of total responsibility, explaining the need for a support network, and training on how to prevent escalation. This stage concludes with the presentation of a therapy roadmap. The next therapeutic task is the formulation and delivery of *the announcement*. This is a semi-formal event, in which parents convey to their child, both by word of mouth and in writing, the changes they have decided to institute in their attitude and behavior. The announcement typifies NVR in its emphasis on resistance rather than control. Preparing for the announcement and its delivery introduces parents to the basic attitude of NVR, in which they: (a) learn to view their resistance as a function of their own readiness, and not of the child's reactions; (b) prepare to cope with the child's reactions without escalating; and (c) learn to focus on changes in their behavior, rather than on immediate improvements in the adult-child. The next task is the constitution of a *support group*. This task can take place parallel to preparation of the announcement. The therapist helps parents rally social support, conducts the meeting with the supporters, and guides the group after the meeting. The next therapeutic stage is the gradual process of *de-accommodation*. Coping with violent, destructive and dangerous behaviors is the first priority all through this process. De-accommodation consists in a series of gradual exposures to diminishing services, infringement of prohibitions and, if necessary, change of living arrangements. The therapist helps the parents set goals, contain their child's reactions and maintain the relationship with the child. The *conclusion stage* is usually open-ended, offering parents the option of returning to therapy for a short period if crises arise.

Chapter 4 (Suicide Threats) presents the NVR approach to suicide threats that, tacitly or overtly, are highly present in families with adult-children. Although the literature on suicide is immense, little has been written on how parents can cope when the child voices a suicide threat. As we shall see, we focus especially on threats that are voiced or intimated as a reaction to the parents' de-accommodation. Parents are helped to cope with those situations by moving from helplessness to presence, from isolation to support, from submission to resistance, from escalation to self-control and from distance to supportive care.

Chapter 5 (Helping Parents of Children and Adolescents at Risk of Failure to Emerge) deals with the precursors of AED in childhood and adolescence. The major risk factors are digital abuse, school refusal, social withdrawal, "tyrannical behaviors" and irresponsible financial behavior. Non-Violent Resistance interventions are described that help parents deal with those conditions.

Chapter 6 (Addressing Entrenched Dependence in Special Contexts) describes how to deal with situations that require adaptations of the protocol described in Chapter 3. Some of these are: emergencies (e.g., psychotic breakdown, suicide attempt or trouble with the police), worrisome conditions that do not yet constitute full-fledged AED, very old parents and the implementation of NVR in a psychiatric ward.

Chapter 7 (Survival Mode: the Adult-Child's Experience), written by Ohad Nahum, describes AED from the adult-child's perspective, and how contact with them (either in the context of a parallel individual therapy or single meeting with the parents' therapist) may enhance the chances of improvement.

The Conclusion points out some of the many questions that require further exploration, such as the etiology and social impact of AED, as well as the efficacy of our intervention. It also expresses the need for courage as a major prerequisite for this process. Adult Entrenched Dependence can induce great fear in parents, adult-children and therapists alike. We see it as one of the virtues of NVR, both in the sociopolitical and family contexts, that it also inspires courage in the meek, the fearful and the oppressed.

AED, the Intervention and Global Diversity

Nonemergence into adulthood and Adult Entrenched Dependence are observed in many cultures. Much work is still needed to understand the interplay of global trends and culture-specific factors in shaping these phenomena (Teo & Gaw, 2010). The same should apply to developing effective culture-specific interventions. Most of our development work was done in the context of our own culture. Although we are certain that members of many other cultures would find it useful, any application of the intervention model presented in this book to a given culture should involve consideration of that culture's specific coming-of-age connotations, symbols and crises.

A Word of Caution

This book is intended as a guide for mental health professionals interested in NVR interventions. Work on AED can be very rewarding but it requires a cautious attitude, as it destabilizes some very entrenched family patterns. We recommend against trying to implement our therapy manual without appropriate background in the mental health professions or without the support of a team.

With Gratitude and Acknowledgment

Looking back on ten years of work, we wish to acknowledge the people whose collaboration, effort and perspective made it possible.

First and foremost are the outstandingly courageous parents, adult-children and extended families who invited us to accompany them through their valley of shadow and fear.

We also wish to thank members of the team who over the years took part in our clinical journey into the uncharted territory of AED: Ohad Nahum, Eli Lebowitz, Yuval Nuss, Amos Spivak, Dana Mor, Efi Nortov, Nevo Pik, Mazal Landes, Noam Israeli, and Uri Nitsan.

Thanks also to the staff at Women's Psychiatric Ward A of the Sheba Medical Center, Ramat Gan, Israel, who during 2013–2014 collaborated with us in working with families of inpatients, and especially Yosef Zohar, Alzbeta Juven Wetzler, Bruria Nussbaum, Sinaya Cohen and Nava Peri. Additionally, we are grateful to Sylvia Tobelem Azulay of the Israel Mental Health Association and to Perah Somech of the Tel Aviv Municipality's social services department for their interest and openness.

We would like to thank the colleagues who over the years collaborated with us in establishing the practice of NVR for AED in their own countries: Peter Jakob in the United Kingdom, Willem Beckers in Belgium, Jan Olthof and Henk Breugem in the Netherlands, Michaela Fried in Austria and Daniel Wulff and Sally St. George in Canada.

Finally we wish to thank Jeffrey Arnett for his inspiring writings, moral support and valuable comments on terminology.

1 The Adult-Child

Functional and Dysfunctional Dependence

Never did a young person's journey to adulthood seem so long and precarious as at the beginning of the twenty-first century. The complexity of choice, uncertainty of outcome, reign of individualism and pressures of competitiveness can become a heavy burden. To many young people, the path to adulthood will at some point seem like a menacing labyrinth.

This book is about families of young people who at some point stop progressing toward psychosocial adulthood. Instead of venturing farther from the parental home, they dig themselves deeper into it. Intimacy is replaced by social networks and work by computer gaming. Biologically, these young people are adults, but psychosocially they are still children. We call them *adult-children*, and the family pattern that evolves around them *entrenched dependence*.

We shall try to understand the family dynamics that perpetuate this condition and present ways to prevent or reverse it. Parents are our potential partners in this process. They are usually the ones who have the motivation and can be helped to jumpstart the arrested development of their adult-child.

Since the early 2000s, we have studied and treated hundreds of families with adult-children or adolescents at risk of becoming such. The sheer numbers of parents who came to us for help indicated a growing problem, which despite its severity often remained hidden behind walls of shame, helplessness and fear.

Adult-children are usually Not in Education, Employment or Training (NEET). Their social ties with peers are minimal. Many have a reversed day/night cycle and are addicted to social or gaming networks. Many spend their waking hours within the home or confined to their rooms. In certain cases, the adult-child locks the door, coming out only at night. Some spend part of their time outside the parental home and go out with friends, but are totally dependent on their parents for physical and financial support. Over the years, even the most outgoing adult-children end up spending most of their lives in seclusion.

Parents of adult-children live in constant worry and anxiety. This preoccupation taxes their sleep, health, work and family life. Marital tensions tend to revolve around the child, with a great deal of finger-pointing. A veil of secrecy surrounds the family. Visitors are often avoided, and contact with family and friends minimized.

The siblings of adult-children are usually independent, and maintain physical or emotional distance from their problematic sibling. They sometimes feel obligated to side with their parents, but are also deeply critical of their over-protectiveness and resent the inordinate amount of attention and resources that the adult-child receives.

The adult-child expects and demands a variety of emotional and material services, such as money, housekeeping or transportation. They also impose special constraints on acceptable parental behavior. These demands are bolstered by declarations of incapacity ("I'm unable to go to school or to work"; "I cannot go out"; "I'm ill!"), blame ("This is your fault!"; "You made me like this!") and threat ("If you don't do this, something awful will happen!"). Those messages are not always explicit. Sometimes, the only explicit demand is to be left alone, but the "leave me alone!" message implies a host of services that enable the adult-child's being left alone. The adult-child's message of incapacity, blame and threat often imbues their claims with an undertone of an inalienable right – a sense of entitlement.

Parents usually react to this discourse with pity, guilt and fear. This attitude is the perfect complement to the adult-child's triad of incapacity, blame and threat. The parents develop a sense of obligation as a counterpart to their child's dysfunction, accommodating the adult-child's ever-increasing needs and expectations. This accommodation deepens the adult-child's helplessness, which in turn intensifies the parents' feeling that they have no option but to continue along the same track (Figure 1). Occasionally, frustration leads a parent to present the

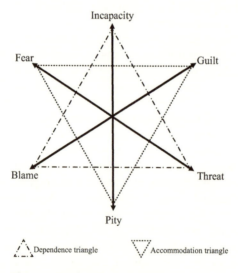

Figure 1 Dysfunctional dependence

adult-child with a set of angry demands. The result is usually an escalation in which the adult-child panics, throws a tantrum or threatens suicide. One of the parents then feels obliged to concede, thus deepening the family's plight. This vicious cycle can persist for years, even decades.

The adult-child's isolation is exacerbated by the parents' aversion to disclose the secret. The family withdraws into itself. The family system thus becomes impervious to external influence.

As our experience with such families grew, we learned that patterns of entrenched dependence appeared in conjunction with a wide variety of clinical conditions (e.g., anxiety disorders, learning disabilities, ADHD, OCD, oppositional-defiant disorder, depression, social phobia, high-functioning autism, anorexia nervosa, schizophrenia or conduct disorder), but in many other cases there was no identifiable pathology. We also learned that many parents in our treatment who succeeded in reducing their accommodation and resisting the demands and attacks in a nonescalatory way achieved significant improvements (Lebowitz et al., 2012). Our interventions did not directly treat the underlying mental disorders but often alleviated them by improving the adult-child's functioning, diminishing distress and increasing the chances that the adult-child would assume more responsibility for their life.

While listening to those parents, we recognized many patterns familiar from our work with families of dysfunctional younger children who were caught in the trap of parental pity, guilt and fear. These parents also alternated between accommodation and angry demands. The chief difference was that, with adult-children, those patterns had become more rigid and extreme, the threats more frightening and the despair more rooted. The family's developmental clock seemed to have stopped, with no way to restart it.

Another marked difference was the parents' deep concern that the adult-child might attempt suicide. This issue was present in a large proportion of the cases we treated and, in the past, had proved a powerful deterrent to any parental initiative. This illustrates the compelling nature of the dependence bond. The adult-child had come to experience the refuge offered by the parents as their only existential option. This feeling of life-threat was markedly less common among parents of younger children.

Individual psychotherapy is often seen by the adult-child either as a threat or as an opportunity for postponing any parental initiatives that might undermine their sense of protection. Usually these adult-children say to their parents, "I don't need treatment!" or "You are the ones who need treatment!" In effect, the adult-child is probably right, not because the parents need help more than the child, but because they are usually the ones who have more of an incentive to seek it.

When we started focusing on adult-children, we were entering uncharted territory, a dark galaxy of isolated home-worlds, each inhabited by a constricted family, trapped in its bubble of despair. It seemed that the family structure had evolved to serve the sole purpose of preserving an adult-child in a fully cloistered ecology.

Many of the adult-children had a plausible psychiatric diagnosis but this could hardly account for the extreme dependence, helplessness, violence, clinging and sense of entitlement they exhibited. The family dynamics we witnessed was highly similar across a wide range of diagnoses, and once the dependence–accommodation cycle was interrupted, the adult-child and the family atmosphere improved markedly, regardless of the diagnosis. Thus, AED seems to be a trans-diagnostic condition. Gradually, we learned that many contemporary cultures have developed derogatory labels for similarly dysfunctional adult-children, such as "boomerang children," "twixters," "adultescents," "NEETs," "KIPPERS" (Kids in Parents' Pockets Eroding Retirement Savings), "parasaito shinguru" ("parasite singles" in Japan), "bamboccioni" or "mammoni" (Italy), "nesthockers" (Germany), "mamma hotel children" (Austria) and Tanguy syndrome (France). These labels suggest that in today's societies coming of age is proving riskier and more difficult. Emerging adulthood theory, formulated at the dawn of the twenty-first century, offered a cross-cultural look at this phenomenon (Arnett, 2000), and hence a good starting point.

The Age of Emerging Adulthood

Many adults born in the 1950s and 1960s are perplexed at the sight of their children in their mid-20s who still live with them or at their expense, flitting between jobs and romantic partners, experimenting freely with unrealistic vocational plans and spending their meagre income on high-end consumer goods. "When I was your age," the parents complain, "I was already married and had two kids"; "When I was 18 I couldn't wait to leave my parents' home." From their perspective, a breach has occurred in the right order of development, threatening to become a chasm between adolescence and adulthood. According to a well-known theory, this gap may represent a new developmental stage, that of *emerging adulthood* (Arnett, 2004). Emerging adulthood is not simply extended adolescence, since it allows for a far wider horizon of exploration away from parental control. Nor is it adulthood, since it does not involve the responsibilities traditionally associated with being an adult. This phase is described as a time for exploring one's identity, professional inclinations and interpersonal relations. It is a time of instability, when abodes shift, and plans are made only to be revised. Emerging adulthood is the life stage of open futures and high hopes, offering the gradually emerging adult the opportunity to free themselves from the chronic unhappiness inherent to many families of origin.

Some observers of emerging adulthood see it as a highly desirable condition. They enthusiastically advocate the right of young (and not-so-young) people to explore their identity and test out multiple jobs and relationships. They see emerging adulthood as a creative response to a confusing postindustrial era. These young people are described in optimistic terms, such as "thriving, struggling and hopeful" (Arnett & Schwab, 2012), or "busy, joyful, stressed – and still dreaming big" (Arnett & Schwab, 2014). Even neurobiology seems to advocate emerging adulthood, with studies suggesting that the structural development of the adolescent and postadolescent brain craves new and varied experience. Hence, emerging adulthood is consistent with brain development and good for the IQ (Steinberg, 2014).

Not unexpectedly, the most enthusiastic advocates of emerging adulthood are emerging adults themselves. As one emerging adult blogger stated: "As I digested emerging adulthood nothing tasted so sweet and fulfilling – like eating an entire cheesecake without any of the guilt or gas. Because we've been told our whole lives to just keep climbing those stairs. Emerging adulthood is what happens when we actually get off the stairs and start exploring — all the dead ends and wrong turns included" (Angone, 2014). Emerging adults enjoy justifying themselves by explaining emerging adulthood theory to their parents. Many parents also welcome emerging adulthood and are ready to support their 20-somethings.

However, there is an underside to all that. For many, the transition to adulthood looks more like a crisis than a period of experimentation. The dysfunctional pattern of dependence we are discussing illustrates this crisis and the failure to resolve it.

In effect, adult-children do not seem to be exploring a new identity. They do not display the energetic trial and error that emerging adults do in terms of habitation, mate selection and plan revisions. Though some may experiment with alternative images of self, this occurs only in phantasy or in the virtual world. They do not explore their own possibilities and are not interested in others, except in their parents, and even then, only as objects of blame or as service providers. AED thus appears to be the other side of the emerging adulthood coin. It is what happens when adulthood fails to emerge.

From Crisis to Failure: the Role of Parental Uncertainty

Emerging adulthood forces today's parents of young adults to play a role for which they have no model and to act in ways that are contrary to their values. When they grew up, young people did not have to be shown out of the family home. On the contrary, they moved out at a rather young age. The average age of marriage for women and men between the end of World War II and the mid-1970s remained stable: 21 for women and 23 for men. By the year 2000, it had risen to 25 and 27, respectively. Today, especially in the middle and upper classes, the comparable figures are 28 and 30, respectively (US Census Bureau, 2018).

According to the traditional parent–child role division, parents hold on to the child and the child tries to break away. Traditionally, the passage to adulthood was articulated as something that happened spontaneously. Children "came of age," "matured," "ripened," "fledged," "seasoned," "flew the nest." Today's parents are far more involved than their own parents were in initiating their children into adulthood. New idioms are needed to express this active role. We talk about "launching" the child and "sending them off." Today the nest can no longer be counted on to empty itself. It often requires proactive emptying.

Many parents of adult-children experience "comparative moments" when they remember the conditions in which they grew up as starker and their transition to adult independence as more abrupt than their children's. Nearly half the parents of emerging adults surveyed in the 2013 Clark University Poll said they gave their 18 to 29 year olds "frequent support when needed" or "regular support for living expenses" (Arnett & Schwab, 2013). When parents were asked about the financial help they had received from their parents, only 14 percent of those parents said they had received either "frequent support" or "regular support for living expenses" when they were in their 20s.

This difference between what today's parents give their children and what they had received from their own is a constant source of ambivalence in parental giving. Time and again parents ask themselves, "Where should I draw the boundary between too little, enough, and too much?" This uncertainty often generates a mixed message, where excessive giving is coupled with "when I was your age" complaints, nagging about the child's dependence, and unrealistic expectations of gratitude and performance.

There are no set guidelines on how to deal with a child who is an emerging adult. There is a multitude of developmental charts and guidelines about when toilet training should start, when girls should reach puberty and what an adolescent's normative cognitive skills comprise. This developmental path stops at 18 and then takes the form of a long fuzzy tunnel, a labyrinth, terminating (with luck) when the child is in their 30s, in some combination of marriage, parenthood, separate habitation and financial independence. Parents of emerging adults do not know what is right and what can be expected. Is it good for my child to live with us? Should I collect rent? Is it still my business to know where they are going and with whom?

This normative vacuum makes today's parents much more vulnerable. To resist inappropriate demands, parents need firm ground to stand upon. Today's parents, however, are in quicksand. The situation becomes even more difficult when they feel anxious, guilty and are not in agreement. When those conditions meet with adjustment difficulties on the child's part, the emergence crisis risks becoming an emergence failure. The struggling adolescent may then grow into an adult-child.

A Realistic Goal: Functional Dependence

Personal independence as an ultimate value is so much a part of the modern worldview that it is difficult to imagine a happy adult life without it. Independence is synonymous with normative adulthood. It is a premise of modern society, closely related to valued notions like authenticity, individuality and freedom. Independence is the culmination of selfhood. In contrast, the notion of dependence is fraught with negative connotations. But this was not always so. In the past, independence was often seen more as an ideal than a normative condition. It was not seen as a hallmark of adulthood.

The view of personal and financial independence as the essential marker of adulthood was fueled by the post–World War II economic boom. Since the late 1940s, the availability of motor cars, credit, mortgages and affordable consumer goods has given young people the feeling that independence is at their fingertips. Since the 1980s, however, the narrative of independence seems under siege. Falling wages, market meltdowns and rising housing costs are making the dream of independence increasingly difficult to realize.

On closer inspection, adulthood cannot be equated with independence. Financial independence from parents almost automatically means dependence on a job market and on the economy that regulates it. Marriage as the traditional marker of independence from one's family of origin actually means a new interdependence between spouses. Even in the booming postwar economy, people had to depend on an employer in order to pay their mortgage. They simply had enough buying power, job security and access to technology to feel independent, while depending. All considered, the full realization of independence as an ideal of total freedom might be closer to eccentricity and marginality than maturity. The completely independent person would probably be also unreliable, as many an abandoned spouse, child or parent would attest.

Indeed, life is a virtually infinite chain of dependencies. Independence is the experience of dependencies that are so reliable that we take them for granted. Any of life's plentiful accidents, disruptions and malfunctions is a reminder of how tenuous one's independence can be. Therefore, our goal is to help parents and adult-children to move not from dependence to independence, but from dysfunctional to functional dependence.

Functional dependence occurs when people are interdependent in a way that sustains their mutual survival, adaptation and well-being. It is the ability to find a middle way between my benefit and that of others, to integrate the giving and taking, helping and being helped.

Many social norms help us distinguish acceptable from unacceptable forms of dependence. For instance, neighbors who occasionally borrow things and then return them, friends who ask for help only after failing to solve a problem on their own and disabled people who need nursing care are universal examples of socially acceptable dependence. Conversely, neighbors who borrow but never lend or friends who try to squeeze us into helping them are examples of unacceptable forms of dependence. The distinction between acceptable and unacceptable forms of dependence is also relevant for parents and children. Even small children know there are things they are expected to do by themselves. As they grow, they learn they are expected to help at home. And when they become adults, the relationship with their parents is expected to become more and more symmetrical. With elderly parents, the direction of dependence may reverse, with the children being expected to support their parents. In AED, these expectations break down. Parents no longer support their child in constructive ways but rather submit to their inappropriate expectations. Adult-children no longer receive appropriate help from their parents but exploit them through passivity, emotional pressure and coercion.

Identifying Dysfunctional Dependence

Learning to distinguish dysfunctional from functional dependence may be the first task for the parents of adult-children. In our work, we have identified questions in five key areas that parents can ask themselves, to help them distinguish between the two.

Do We Have a Time Perspective? Can We Strive toward a Horizon of Better Functioning?

For six years, Bill (28) had lived in university dorms, finished a master's degree in history and worked part-time as an academic assistant. When his application to a PhD program was rejected, he was devastated. He moved back into his parents' home and spent most of his time sleeping or ruminating about his failure. One day, his parents, Sheila and Jack, saw him engrossed in building a Lego tower. Glad to see him doing something productive for change, they pulled out of storage all his childhood assembly games and placed them on a shelf in the living room. Bill started spending more and more time in the living room, building Lego cities. He seemed to have lost interest in his friends but occasionally agreed to accompany his parents when they went shopping or to visit their own friends. A year went by with no change in Bill's condition.

When Bill's parents came to us, they were deeply concerned, but Jack put the best face on the situation. He said that his son seemed more active and less secluded. "Yes," said Sheila, "but would it be right to insist that he come out of his room to greet our guests? Or shall we leave him be? He's a grown man after all."

Parental adaptation to a child's peculiarities can be helpful, if directed at a horizon of better functioning. Bill's parents seemed to have lost that orientation. The father saw Bill playing with Lego for days on end as a good sign. The mother referred to Bill as "a grown man," but only to justify his being allowed to remain undisturbed in his room. These parents were accommodating Bill's childish behavior. When they saw him playing with Lego, they made his assembly games available. Had they forgotten that until recently Bill had been living, studying and working on his own? Bill's parents cared for Bill as they would have cared for a child. They brought out his toys, cooked for him, took him to visit their friends and enjoyed seeing him build Lego cities. It seemed imperative to reintroduce a sense of time and a horizon of functioning into this situation.

We use several questions, messages and metaphors to reorient parents regarding time. One question that may prove helpful is "Where do you see yourselves in 10 years' time?" We try to help the parents focus on their advancing age. Bill's parents were 58 and 53, so the therapist asked them to imagine themselves at 68 and 63. The discussion made it clear that at some point in the future, no matter what their son's condition, they would have to relinquish their protective role.

Launching is the process whereby the parents give up their responsibility for the growing child. Instead of asking "What can I do for my child?" they ask "What should I stop doing for my child?"

To illustrate to parents how launching occurs, we often use the story of the eagle's nest, which we learned from one of the fathers in our treatment. Eagles' nests are rough frames, filled with soft materials like grass, leaves and feathers, and harder ones like twigs. As the fledglings grow, the parent begins to dismantle the nest, first removing the soft materials, and eventually also the hard ones, so the fledglings realize that it is time for them to leave.

A clear time perspective is a major criterion in distinguishing functional support from dysfunctional accommodation. It is common wisdom that "one should provide fishing-rods rather than fish." This saying helps distinguish accommodation from support. Accommodation is not only unhelpful but damaging. It all but guarantees that the child will not put up the effort or develop the skills necessary for better functioning. Parental accommodation may even create the paradoxical effect of deterring the child from making an effort, lest the parents come to the conclusion that their services are no longer needed. A study of anxious children who refused therapy found that many of these children refused to go to treatment because they feared that, if they did, the parents would stop accommodating their fears (Lebowitz et al., 2014).

When parents develop a time perspective and look forward to a horizon of better functioning, they can ask themselves "Does this service that I provide promote my child's capacity to function?" Asking this question is a necessary step in countering dysfunctional dependence.

At this point, however, doubts often arise as to whether the child is at all capable of independent functioning. Parents may then invoke the adult-child's diagnosis and their own bitter history of failures and disappointments. This focus engenders a pessimism that impedes their ability to envision a horizon of better functioning. A helpful therapeutic reaction to the emergence of these paralyzing concerns is to engage the parents in a thought experiment. They are asked to imagine two families, each with a child who has a severe mental illness. In the first family, the parents decide that, since their child is ill, it is pointless to make demands, set boundaries or raise expectations. They treat the child as an invalid and resign themselves to their fate. They put up with aggravation and violence, which they attribute to the child's illness. They incur the anger of their other children and reduce contacts with their extended family and friends, because their social network does not understand how debilitated their child is.

In the second family, the parents decide that, although their child is ill, there are still clear boundaries and obligations. They defend themselves and their other children against violence and coercion. They focus on whatever functional strengths the child does have, as indicative of possible improvement in weaker areas. They limit the services that they offer in areas in which they believe the child can cope.

Then the therapist asks the parents to imagine those two families five years later. What do they expect their situation and the child's condition to be? At some point, the therapist may add their own conclusion: "I don't know what the upper limit to your child's functioning capacity is. It may be this high [drawing a waist high imaginary line] or this high [drawing an imaginary line above the head]. What I know, however, is that your child's functioning level at present is this high [drawing an ankle high imaginary line]."

Do We Live As Persons in Our Own Right? How Can We Recover Our Presence?

Many parents of adult-children believe that the therapy is not at all about them. Were it not for the child's refusal of treatment, they would not be in a therapist's office. They are here for the child's sake, not for their own. Actually, in many of these families, parents have lost sight of their own needs and wants, seeing them as negligible compared to those of the child.

Joseph (54) and Sandra (50) came to see us about their son, Kevin (25), who finished high school six years ago and has lived with them ever since. He sleeps all day, stays up all night and works only rarely. Kevin would go out at night and, when returning, wake up his parents by wandering around the house, cooking, watching TV and sometimes entertaining friends. He often took their car and used their credit card without permission. He abused his mother, locking her in the house twice, when she refused to give him money.

The thought of returning home after work filled Sandra with panic. Joseph worked at home and complained that Kevin interrupted him inconsiderately. Sandra cooked for him and did his laundry. Joseph scheduled and took him to the doctor and paid his parking tickets. Kevin would often come into the living room when his parents were watching TV and take the car keys without a word. If Sandra dared protest or even ask when he would bring back the car, he would ignore her. She sobbed, "It's as if I were invisible." Joseph said that talking to his son was like speaking to a lamppost. The therapist began to list some of the parents' basic unmet needs, such as sleep, quiet, safety and respect. As the therapist asked the parents to think about those aspects of the relationship, Joseph interrupted him, saying, "But listen, we're not here for what *we* need. This isn't about *us*, it is about Kevin."

The process of parental effacement is sometimes apparent in gradual changes in the distribution of living space. In late adolescence, the adult-child usually occupies a single room in the parental home. As years go by, the adult-child begins to take over the living room and then other rooms, using them to store their things. As parents become frail and less mobile, they often end up confined to one small room, with their child occupying the rest of the house. In one of our cases, a 25-year-old man raised two large dogs inside his parents' house. When his mother complained that the dogs were damaging the furniture and soiling the house, he fenced in about two thirds of the house, claiming it as his territory. When she said that she could not stand the dirt, he told her she was free to clean while he walked the dogs.

Parents sometimes lose not only their space but also their social life, leisure and even the connection to their own feelings. The child monopolizes their attention. They constantly ask, "How can we get him to find a job?" "How do we get her out of her room and into the living room?" "What can we do to make him socialize?" "How can we get her to go to therapy?" "How can we motivate him?" "How can we make her feel less anxious, have more self-esteem, be happy?"

To start a process of positive change, parents must move from effacement to presence. Presence is engendered when parents behave in ways that convey the message, "I am here and I'll stay here. I am here not only for you but also for myself." We tell parents that the greatest gift they can give their child is that of their regained presence, as people with needs and feelings. The parents come out of their effacement when they declare, "I have needs, therefore I am!" A useful metaphor is the instruction that flight attendants give before take-off: When parents need to use an oxygen mask, they should put their own mask on before putting one on their child. When parents prioritize their need for sleep, respect, safety and well-being, they become better able to care both for themselves and for their child. Prioritizing certain parental needs not only enhances the parent's ability to care, it also gives children of all ages a critically needed model of self-care.

The parents' habits of self-effacement often become obvious in therapy, as the parents reply to every therapeutic suggestion by predicting the child's reaction. It is as if they had no right to any position that their child would find unacceptable. Sometimes, parents are so used to thinking their child's thoughts instead of their own, that they even answer the therapist's suggestions or comments in the child's voice:

THERAPIST: One of the tools we use in our work is the announcement. It is a text that you deliver in a quasi-formal manner to your son, declaring that you have decided to reject his unacceptable behaviors.
FATHER: What do you mean? Is it something we say to him?
THERAPIST: You read it to him from a written page.
MOTHER: I don't care what's on your stupid page!
THERAPIST: Excuse me?
MOTHER: I mean, that's what he would say. He won't listen.

Another way in which parents enact their effacement in the session is by repeatedly asking "What do we say when he ... ?" "How do I react when she ... ?" We call this *negative hypnosis*. The parents are so focused on the adult-child's behavior that they lose sight of any option that is not an immediate reaction to the adult-child's cue.

One suggestion that many parents find helpful is to change the focus from "What can I do for my child?" to "What can I *not* do for them?" Parents develop the courage to tell the adult-child that they will no longer perform some services. These responses are then discussed, rehearsed or role-played in therapy. Thinking seriously about what parents cannot do for their child is a way of recovering their presence as persons. This is crucial in moving from dysfunctional to functional dependence.

Another direction we often take, when trying to help awaken parents from their reactive trance, is to change the focus from "What can I do for my child?" to "What kind of person do I want to be, as a parent?" We use these questions to explore with parents how they see their role in their adult-child's life, and what alternative views of that role can be considered. Anchoring on what kind of person the parent wants to be, helps them regain a sense of presence and discover what they should do, not as a reaction to the child's behavior, but as a consequence of their own wishes.

Have I Bowed to a Fate of Total Sacrifice for My Child? Can I Dare and Recommit Myself to Wellness?

Frank and Sarah came to see us about their daughter, Adriana (34). Until she was 24, Adriana had seemed like a typical emerging adult. She completed high school, earned a degree from a reputable drama school and began performing in professional theatre productions. She was socially active and had had a long-term romantic relationship. Then she began washing her hands compulsively and spending inordinate amounts of time in the toilet. She developed a persistent fear of being contaminated by her own feces. Those worries became the center of her life. She gave up her job, withdrew from social activities and spent most of her waking hours in sanitation rituals associated with her toilet visits. She flatly refused any form of treatment.

Adriana's mother, Sarah, became increasingly involved in Adriana's rituals. When Sarah wouldn't do what Adriana wanted, Adriana would become verbally and physically abusive. Frank looked on helplessly as family life disintegrated. Six years after Adriana's disorder erupted, Sarah moved out of the bedroom that she shared with her husband to sleep on a sofa outside Adriana's room, so that she would be available for her nighttime rituals. Adriana's demands for Sarah's time and attention reached the point that Adriana would threaten suicide if her mother left her alone for more than a few hours. Frank immersed himself in his work and tried to spend as little time as possible at home, occasionally spending the night in his office. He sought comfort with his daughter Silvia, Adriana's elder sister, who had distanced herself from the family. To accommodate Adriana, the parents spent large sums of money on wholesale quantities of toilet paper, heating gas, water and soap. As Frank confided to us, every time he saw Adriana's name flash on his phone screen, his pulse would accelerate and he would feel a pain in his chest.

Sarah withdrew from the therapy after a couple of sessions, arguing that Adriana needed her presence at home. Frank and Silvia continued attending together. After several months of careful deliberation, including consultations with members of the extended family, it was suggested that Sarah be eased out of her role as Adriana's servant, by having her (Sarah) leave the home for a few weeks, and replacing her with nursing staff and some members of the extended family.

Frank and Silvia invited Sarah to a crucial therapy session, together with five other family members. Sarah agreed to attend that session, among other reasons, because she felt responsible for whatever decision was about to be taken regarding Adriana. During that session, Sarah agreed to the plan. The next day, a group of 10 people, including Frank, Silvia, Sarah's brother, three other relatives, a psychiatrist, two nurses and the family's therapist entered the family home. The psychiatrist told Sarah that the nurses would take up her cleaning duties. Sarah, who had agreed to the move "under duress," took five minutes to pack up and leave, ending a decade of abject servitude. Within a week, Sarah's mood, appetite and sleep had improved. She resumed her hobbies and made up for lost time. Frank and Sarah moved together into a rented apartment. While the medical team and other relatives took turns looking after Adriana and helping her adjust to a new reality, Frank and Sarah experienced a marital comeback. At the end of the therapy, they described it as a second honeymoon. After six months, the couple returned home to an entirely new situation. Sarah did not take up her old role as provider of inappropriate services for her daughter. Adriana's OCD receded. She began taking medications and attended psychotherapy. Sarah said: "It's incredible! Adriana survived and I can breathe!"

Parents of adult-children often resort to counseling only when their suffering becomes unbearable. Even then, they often say they would be willing to go on suffering, if only their child would get well. Our counselling process begins with an attempt to turn the tables on this self-sacrificing stance. To be able to let the child go, the parents must release their own suffering and recommit themselves to wellness as a supreme life value that includes safety, health, social contacts and the right to happiness. Dysfunctional dependence is perpetuated when these values are subordinated to appeasing a child's anxiety. We once asked a self-sacrificing mother, "If you knew that striving to live a fuller life was the best contribution you could make both to yourself and to your child – would you do it?"

She answered: "If it would help her, I would do even that!"

But the sacrifice that comes with carrying a dysfunctionally dependent child on one's back is not just any pain that will go away because we wish it would. Accommodating parents see no other choice but pay for the child's survival with their sleep, peace of mind, marital life and comfort. The self-sacrificing parent embodies a model of total devotion that is admired in many cultures. Such parents would feel worthless were they to relinquish that role. Self-sacrifice rests on the assumption that only the parent can save the child. Only the parent understands the child's needs, feels the child's distress and is capable of the devotion needed to take care of that child. Sometimes, guilt feeds into self-sacrifice. Some parents feel that they must atone for old mistakes. Conversely, they fear they will feel unbearable guilt if they give up that role. They might then feel like the parents of Hansel and Gretel, who abandoned their children in the woods. So long as these assumptions remain unchallenged, the dysfunctional dependence bond will be maintained. To dissolve that bond, we deploy a systematic process of persuasion.

Self-sacrificing parents are helped to understand the profound connection between their accommodation to the child's demands and expectations, and the perpetuation of the child's dysfunction. This conversation, usually accompanied by some initial experiments in reducing accommodation, takes place at the beginning of treatment. It is often helpful to cite research data and clinical experience on the role of parental accommodation in exacerbating the symptoms and dysfunction. Parents are also asked to imagine or remember times when the adult-child functioned better. As parents take initial steps of de-accommodation, the impact of these steps is carefully evaluated. Almost always the adult-child demonstrates some adaptability, even if under protest. This helps mitigate the inexorable logic of self-sacrifice.

Parents are also asked to imagine what would happen if, for reasons beyond their control, their support became unavailable to the child. Some self-sacrificing parents share with us their phantasies of falling ill or being hospitalized, which would force them out of their roles as compulsory saviors. In this way, it gradually becomes possible to refute the idea that nobody but the self-sacrificing parent can rescue the child. On the contrary, continuing the self-sacrifice is now viewed as the guarantee that the adult-child will never get better. This conversation leads to the suggestion that the adult child's best hope would be that the parents relinquish their self-sacrificing role. Many parents are intrigued by this possibility.

This may pave the way to the special strategy of "honorable reprieve." With the help of a support group of relatives and friends, the self-sacrificing parent is temporarily removed from the field. The other parent and the support group make it clear that they will handle the challenge in a humane, and at the same time resolute, manner. It may be important to stress that it would take an entire group of people to perform what one self-sacrificing parent does. There is honor in this acknowledgment. The presence of a chorus of encouraging and committed voices, seconded by professionals, often allows the self-sacrificing parent to make a bold dash toward a much deserved respite. In this way, the whole ecology of dysfunctional dependence may be changed in one fell swoop.

Barry was 16 when he gradually stopped going to school. Highly anxious and a perfectionist, he began skipping school after barely passing an exam in math, a subject in which he had excelled. At first, he would refuse to go to school on exam days, and then started staying home regularly. His father, Mark, offered to drive him to school and to talk to his teachers. For a time, Barry seemed to cooperate, but one day the two had a fierce argument and Barry physically pushed Mark out of his room. The incident horrified Barry's mother, Alice, who sided with her son, accusing Mark of escalating Barry's anxiety. At that point, Barry stopped going to school altogether, refused to talk to his father and secluded himself in his room. Alice became Barry's around-the-clock caregiver. She would bring meals into his room and was constantly on call, in case Barry needed reassurance.

Three months later, Barry promised to go back to school, on the condition that his parents would allow him to move into a guest suite they occasionally rented out. Alice and Mark agreed. Barry moved into the suite but after attending school for only two days he came home and declared that he was not going back. Alice quit her job in order to become Barry's full-time caretaker. She would clean his suite, hold long daily conversations with him, cook special dishes for him and serve them in his room. Barry began demanding that she divorce Mark, arguing that his father had always demeaned and emotionally traumatized him. The guest suite Barry moved into included a bathroom, a mini kitchen and refrigerator, which, combined with his mother's dedicated room service enabled him to completely cloister himself in his rooms. He cut off all his ties to the surrounding world, apart from his mother. This went on for a year.

In the first therapy session, Mark broke down in tears, saying he had forgotten what his son looked like. Despite all her accommodation to Barry, Alice knew that Barry and his father had been quite close, at least until the moment when Mark opposed Barry's school avoidance. Given the breakdown in the father–son relationship, however, Alice saw herself as Barry's only remaining link to life.

The first three months of therapy focused on understanding how Alice's accommodation was only enabling Barry's self-isolation. Although she could understand that being at Barry's beck and call was not helping him, she said she could not act otherwise. She felt she was Barry's oxygen line and that without her he would suffocate. At the same time, she had come to see Barry as disabled. She was asked to imagine what would happen to Barry if she fell ill. She replied that for as long as she could stand, she would devote herself to her son.

At this juncture Mark recalled a crucial family memory. At the age of 12, Barry underwent an episode of deep anxiety. He began sleeping with his parents, and ultimately convinced Alice to sleep in his room at night. After several months, Alice's mother, who lived abroad, was diagnosed with terminal cancer. Alice left the country to tend to her mother in her final month. Barry reacted to Alice's absence in a very positive way. Upon returning home, she discovered that, while she was gone, Barry had gone back sleeping alone in his room, and was helping Mark with shopping, cleaning and cooking. The two even went out on a three-day fishing trip. Barry was very proud of his achievements.

This memory helped moderate Alice's view of herself as helping her son through self-sacrifice. It became clear that so long as Barry was allowed to live in his suite and was catered for by his mother, his chances of coping would remain extremely low. Alice reflected that perhaps she needed another emergency to make her unavailable to Barry.

Mark's two brothers and their wives, as well as two of Alice's closest friends, were invited to the next session. All the participants knew how positively Alice's enforced absence during her mother's illness had affected Barry some years earlier. All agreed that Barry's protective haven was actually a place of stagnation, where he would only become less and less functional. Alice agreed but said that, so long as she was around, she could not keep herself from running to Barry's rescue. One of Alice's friends made an exciting offer: The two of them would take the three-week trek in the Himalayas they had always dreamt of doing. The trip would require gradual adaptation to high-altitude conditions, and there would be no mobile phone service. Everyone in the room approved of the idea, agreeing that both Barry and Alice deserved it.

After a month of preparations, Alice and her friend were off to the Himalayas. Alice refrained from giving Mark any suggestions or instructions about how to handle Barry. She also resolved to be unreachable by phone from the moment of departure. Over several sessions, Mark, his brothers and the therapist contemplated a plan for a "nonescalating invasion" of Barry's territory. Barry finally agreed to let one of his uncles into his room. The uncle stayed with him for one hour, then Mark was allowed to come in. Initially, Barry avoided eye contact with his father and responded to all his questions in monosyllables, but over the few next days went shopping with him and took an active part in housekeeping.

When Alice returned from her trek, she found Barry enrolled in an intensive computer programming course. Several months later, he moved out of his parents' home and into a small apartment they helped him rent. His next step was to enlist in the army, where he served as a computer programmer. Barry remained deeply offended by what he perceived as his father forcing him out of his room. He eventually severed all contact with Mark but never relapsed into his dysfunctional dependence on his parents.[1]

How Are We Encouraging Our Child's Entitlement?

Lyanne (60) came to see us because of her difficulties with her son, Larry (23). Larry had dropped out of high school at age 17 and spent the past six years living in a basement room in the house his mother and stepfather shared. He had worked for half a year at a computer retail store but quit because he believed he deserved better pay. After discovering that other jobs paid even less, he began spending most of his time in his room or hanging out with a few friends. He slept during the day and went out at night. Lyanne did all his cooking and laundry and cleaned up after him. She even replenished his supply of after-shave. She would keep tabs on the amount of aftershave left in his bottle and made sure that he always had enough. Larry had never bothered to ask her to do this; he felt entitled and Lyanne complied. So when the local drugstore stopped carrying Larry's favorite brand of aftershave and Lyanne was unable to keep him supplied, Larry was irate. Lyanne felt a tinge of guilt. She thought his expectations and her sense of obligation were natural, because of his emotional difficulties.

---

[1] During the coronavirus lockdown we received a message from the parents: Barry had reestablished contact with his father, after a lapse of 10 years.

Entitlement is not only an individual attitude but an interpersonally constructed reality. Among the services that entitled adult-children expect from their parents are laundry, cleaning, meals, money, unlimited access to their car, absolute privacy, and the right to reassurance and comfort. The darker side of entitlement is the "right" to blame and abuse the parents when they fail to live up to expectations or for allegedly having caused the child's dysfunction in the first place. The accommodating parents of adult-children work hard to keep them satisfied. Parents in their 60s and 70s still cook, clean and shop for children in their 20s and 30s. They provide them not only with spending money but sometimes with regular monthly "salaries," they schedule their doctor's appointments and drive them to make sure they arrive on time. They also work hard to conceal their child's problematic behaviors from their friends and other members of the family.

Entitlement is often maintained by the shared assumption that the adult-child is absolutely unable to function on their own. Attempts to question the adult-child's expectations usually result in threatened or actual violence by the adult-child, feelings of guilt in the parents and high anxiety on both sides. Tragically, parents who believe they are the child's last and only support are often correct. Like Atlas, they end up carrying the child's world on their shoulders, convinced disaster would follow if they flinched.

In a more functionally dependent relationship, the link between disability and service is far more flexible. There is an expectation that the dependent's functioning will improve when services are reduced. Even where the disability is a physical given, there is a continuous search for ways to compensate for it. Loosening entitled expectations and recreating a sense of alternatives is therefore a necessary step in the gradual transformation of dysfunctional into functional dependence.

One way is to help parents relinquish their belief that they are the child's only possible support. A helpful strategy is to introduce the parents to a rehabilitation or financial expert. This can help regardless of the adult-child's inclination to cooperate. For instance, with adult-children who squander money, the parents can bring in a financial expert to examine their financial management and advise them on how to balance their budget. Any further provision of money is then made contingent on the expert's report. If the child refuses to cooperate, the parents will feel much more justified to withhold funds. This attitude is widely accepted in society: When a person, business or state become insolvent, help is made contingent on a recovery plan, in which the debtor's economic performance is closely monitored. Since the parents are not in a good position to monitor the adult-child's expenses, the introduction of a third party can provide both sides with a guarantee of fairness, without parental invasion of the adult-child's personal sphere. Many parents we worked with were able to change their giving patterns when a financial expert was introduced. The adult-child would often protest but eventually adapt. With some adult-children, the introduction of a rehabilitation expert, even if not conducive to immediate progress, may start a process of separating the child's needs from the parents' services. In a study of adult-children with HFASD, we showed how helping parents to envisage the eventual transfer of their child to supported housing began preparing them to gradually reduce their accommodation and, as a result, the child's entitlement (Golan et al., 2018).

Another strategy we use to loosen entitled expectations is to reconnect the nuclear family to its wider social network. As the relational patterns of AED develop, they tend to deepen the family's isolation, thereby weakening the parents' ability to cope. Creating a support group of relatives and friends allows the parents to reduce their exclusive involvement with the adult-child. The adult-child, in turn, is offered an experience of decentralized support. Luckily, external supporters are less accommodating of the child's expectations, thus creating better conditions for a more functional dependence.

Alex (64) and Diana (56) came to see us about their daughter Amy (28), who had spent most of the past four years ruminating about her physical condition. The blinds in her room were permanently shut. The walls were covered with sticky notes and printouts with affirmations containing messages of self-encouragement (e.g., "there is light at the end of the tunnel!") and threats against her parents (e.g., "she made me ill, she will pay!"). The printouts were medical test results. According to Amy, her chronic stomachaches prevented her from working, studying, leaving home and forming social relationships. The pains also kept her from eating properly, so she was underweight. Amy believed that the pains were chronic sequelae to the psychiatric medications her mother had made her take. The medications had been prescribed after Amy developed paranoid symptoms, a host of incapacitating fears and repeatedly threatened suicide. She attributed her symptoms to a horrible secret she had been harboring for years and could not disclose. Her symptoms appeared between the ages of 18 and 24, when she still seemed like many other emerging adults. She had completed a BA in biology, lived on campus, dated and held a job. At 24, however, she began dedicating all her resources to a single project: finding medical evidence that her psychiatric medications had caused her suffering. She had taken every conceivable medical test, tried all available therapies, read the medical literature, corresponded with internationally renowned researchers and, with time, became somewhat of an authority on the gastric effects of psychiatric medication. She held her parents accountable for her condition – they had made her take the medication and were therefore responsible for remedying it. She expected her mother to be constantly available to discuss her condition and treatments. She demanded that her parents cover all costs of her sometimes abstruse and expensive treatments, as well as

to drive her to her numerous medical appointments. Amy overreacted whenever her parents tried to leave the house, even for a few hours, wondering how
they could enjoy themselves while she was in agony. Diana was in continuous
anguish because of Amy. Every night, she would wake up several times to
check if her daughter was still breathing.

According to her medical tests, Amy was physically healthy. Alex and Diana
attributed her distress to a mental disorder. In the past Amy had admitted to
mental problems. She attended psychotherapy twice a week for several years
and then stopped, claiming that therapy had helped her resolve her mental
issues, leaving only her physical health to deal with.

The parents spent inordinate amounts of money on Amy's treatments each
month. Desperate to see her leave home, Alex had once deposited $25,000 in
her bank account, hoping she would use the money to rent an apartment. During
the sessions Alex and Diana understood that the critical issue was not whether
Amy was truly ill, but whether her illness justified her sense of entitlement.
They decided to tell her:

1. That they fully understood she was suffering.
2. That they did not feel responsible for her suffering or for the way she
   conducted her life.
3. That they were willing to help her with any constructive plan, but that her
   illness was something she would have to take care of by herself.
4. That they would no longer drive her to doctors' appointments, discuss her
   medical condition with her, help her do research on the Internet or pay for
   her treatments.
5. That given her age and theirs, she should move out of the family home into
   her own apartment. They set a three-month deadline.

Amy's initial reaction to these statements was a veiled suicide threat: "OK,
I've already said goodbye to everybody!" The therapist had convened
a meeting of Amy's relatives and friends ahead of time to discuss ways to
support her parents. Expecting Amy to threaten suicide, they already had
a plan. The parents notified some of the supporters in the group, each of
whom then contacted Amy and conveyed to her the following general message,
each in their own way: "Your parents told us about their decision, and that you
said you had already said goodbye to everybody. I want you to know that I care
for you very much and don't want to say goodbye. I'm saying 'hello,' and 'let's
be in touch,' and 'let's see how I can help you.'"

Amy made no more suicide threats. A couple of weeks following the
announcement, Amy contacted her father, to whom she had not spoken for
more than a year, saying: "I understand you want to throw me out of the house
in three months. Are you going to help me find an apartment?" The parents
ignored Amy's entitled tone but informed the supporters that Amy was willing
to search for a place to live. From that moment on, Amy enjoyed the support of

the group. A couple of family friends helped her find an apartment. Her uncle helped with the lease. An aunt took her shopping for household items. Her sister and brother-in-law helped her with the actual move and kept her company for the first two days. It turned out that Amy had also a few old friends with whom she reconnected.

Two weeks after Amy moved out she called her mother and tried a new strategy to reinvolve her in the old quest for remedy. "Mom," she said enthusiastically, "we need to take a systemic approach to my problem here. Everyone we know can join hands to find the therapy that will make me feel better." This was already an improvement, a proposal rather than a demand. The mother answered, "You are right, we do need a systemic approach. Why don't you talk to Aunt Giselle about it?" Amy called her aunt and tried to get her help in finding some new therapy for her stomach problem. The aunt replied, "I'm sorry dear, I'd really like to help you but I'm afraid I don't understand much about these things." Amy did not insist. Since this is not a fairy tale with a happy ending, we are not claiming that Amy's problems were solved. However, clear options were opened for the creation of a more functional dependence.

Are We Being Coerced? Blackmailed? Exploited?

Perhaps the most blatant characteristic of entrenched dependence is its coercive and exploitative nature. Parents are not only induced to comply through empathy and compassion for the sufferings of their adult-child but are sometimes forced to do so by a blend of aggression, emotional blackmail and outright exploitation. Direct physical violence is most patent in childhood and adolescence, or when the parents are elderly and often defenseless. Many parents told us that their adult-children had been very violent toward them during childhood and adolescence, but calmed down as they matured. However, it is not infrequent that the parents' attempts to de-accommodate triggers new outbursts of violence. More commonly, the violence that the child threatened is against the self, as in threats of suicide. Many parents are surprised when we tell them that suicide threats should always be resisted, since they refer to an extremely violent act that would destroy both the child's and the parents' lives. There are additional forms of stark emotional blackmail. Adult-children threaten to cut off all relations with their parents, disclose their parents' secrets, sell their own property (which they had received from parents or grandparents) or run away from home (a threat more frequent in adolescence). Alternatively, the adult-child remains in bed, stops eating or taking medication, and shows signs of emotional collapse. Blackmailing in those cases is evident if the adult-child blames the parents for their collapse. Even then, many adult-children seem not to be depressed when they converse with friends by phone, or come out of bed at night to eat clandestinely.

While working with parents, it is important to call out violence, blackmail and exploitation. This must not be done in an indignant tone but as a statement of fact. Our therapy encourages parents to reduce their services, and at the same time resist violence, blackmail and exploitation. To this end, the object of resistance must be explicitly named. So long as parents persist in euphemizing their child's behaviors, they may remain helpless.

Entrenched Dependence from Childhood to Adulthood

Entrenched dependence does not emerge out of nowhere in early adulthood. It almost invariably evolves from relational patterns that appear in childhood and adolescence. This evolution helps explain why parents of adult-children sought our help. Haim Omer has written several books on families where children displayed highly problematic behaviors either from an "externalizing" (e.g., violence, impulsiveness, risk behaviors, substance abuse or delinquency) or an "internalizing" kind (e.g., anxiety, obsessive-compulsive disorder, social withdrawal or computer addiction). He had developed NVR to help the parents of those children overcome their own problematic reactions of hitting out or giving in. As an alternative, parents were taught to avoid escalation while tenaciously resisting the child's problematic behaviors (Omer, 2004b, in press). As NVR developed into new areas, we came to conceptualize it as a way of helping parents to develop an *anchoring function*, which allows them to resist the destructive forces that threaten to sweep away the child and the family (Omer et al., 2013). Those ideas attracted considerable public attention. NVR societies[2] were founded in many countries, culminating in five international conferences (London, Antwerp, Munich, Malmoe and Tel Aviv) in addition to many local events that attracted thousands of participants.[3] A growing number of parents to adults approached us with problems similar to those for which NVR had originally gained recognition. We noticed two recurring themes: the behaviors displayed by their adult-children were similar to those of younger children whose parents we had treated, and the present interactive patterns between the parents and the adult-child had been manifest in the past. We thus concluded that most adult-children whose parents we saw were probably grown-up versions of the children in our previous studies. Entrenched dependence, then, seemed to be a continuum, extending from childhood through adolescence and into adulthood.

Our studies with children and adolescents had shown that the effects of NVR interventions seemed to endure beyond the short term (see Omer, 2004b, in press;

---

[2] The approach and the societies sometimes include the acronym NA (New Authority; Omer, 2011).

[3] The extensive bibliography that accumulated on NVR and NA in various languages can be found at www.Haimomer-NVR.com

Omer & Lebowitz, 2016, for a review).The reason for this was probably that parents had come out of their original passivity and isolation, managed to avoid escalating, stopped accommodating, and learned to resist violence, blackmail and exploitation. There are, of course, differences in family atmosphere, depth of parental despair, amount of shame, and fear of consequences in our work with children and adult-children. Those differences demand special consideration. We have found that therapists working in isolation will often feel too insecure to deal with the potentially explosive cases of adult-children. Thus, whereas the treatment of children and adolescents may be conducted by single therapists, treating the parents of adult-children usually requires a team. The parents' therapist may need the help and backing of a psychiatrist, social worker, financial consultant or rehabilitation expert. Professional support is required, if only to gain the courage to take action. It is the rare therapist who does not lose their peace of mind when confronted with parents who are in a panic about their adult-child's extreme reactions. It takes courage to continue helping parents maintain non-escalating resistance in the face of dire threats. This courage is not born in the therapist's lonely heart it is a product of teamwork. Just as the parents need a supporting network to anchor themselves and stabilize their child, the therapist needs their own network to provide the necessary stability, security and backing. We therefore think that the ideal treatment setting for dealing with adult-children is that of a mental health or rehabilitation clinic with a multidisciplinary staff. As a minimum, we would recommend that therapists treating the parents of adult-children should have the benefit of a group for discussion and mutual supervision, and the possibility of obtaining specialized support where needed.

The relational pattern of entrenched dependence is maintained by the interlocking beliefs, expectations, emotions and acts of parents and their adult-children. Both sides firmly believe in the adult-child's incapacity to function and in the parents' incapacity to withstand the adult-child's pressure. The adult-child's distress elicits concessions that arise from parental guilt, pity and fear. Every now and then, the relationship is punctuated by bouts of frustration and anger, leading to ineffective demands by the parents and fierce accusations and threats by the adult-child. Far from weakening the dysfunctional bond, these outbursts reinforce it, for parents often live in fear of their recurrence. Each inadequate parental service reinforces both the adult-child's feelings of incapacity and the parents' habits of accommodation. Secrecy and social isolation further reinforce the dysfunctional pattern. The more isolated the family, the more intractable the bond of dysfunctional dependence. As this chapter was being written, a mother came to one of us and said, "I am here because my daughter dropped out of school when she was 14 and has not left the house since." When the therapist asked how old the daughter was, the mother replied, "Forty."

Although the dysfunctional bond involves both the adult-child and the parents, the options for change are far from symmetrical. There is an enormous difference in the willingness of both parties to engage in the process of change. Simply put, the child, of whatever age, wishes to maintain the protective shield that the parents provide, while the parents want the child to grow up and be functional. In the past, many therapists assumed that the parents also wished to maintain the dependence bond because of their own subconscious needs. We believe this assumption to be unfounded. Parents maintain their protective stance not because they want to do so, but because they see no alternative. When given the means and support to limit their accommodation, they usually do. In contrast, seldom do inveterate dysfunctional adult-children willingly take the bold steps toward more autonomous functioning. Left to themselves, they tend to cling to their course of avoidance.

The great majority of parents we worked with had previously sought professional help. The results, however, were disappointing for one of the following reasons: the adult-child refused therapy; the adult-child agreed to individual therapy, but AED persisted; parents were advised to show unconditional acceptance; or parents were advised to be tough.

The Adult-Child Refuses Therapy

In our experience, most adult-children refuse therapy. Sometimes, they refuse to attend even a single evaluation session. This intransigence sinks the parents in deep helplessness. Psychiatrists and psychotherapists often tell them, "Your child is a grown-up. If he doesn't want to come, there is nothing I can do." Parents usually try to convince the child of the need for therapy. Their first question to us is often, "How can we make him understand that he needs therapy?" This is a futile endeavor, because therapy that is the result of the parents' nagging is often doomed to fail. In addition, in their eagerness to get the child treated, parents may be tempted to make problematic concessions. Finally, parent-initiated therapy may give the adult-child the leverage to make a new threat: "If you act like this, I'll leave therapy!"

The Adult-Child Agrees to Therapy, but AED Persists

There are different paths by which individual therapy may stabilize the problem situation instead of leading to improved functioning. For instance, therapy may give the adult-child a comfortable way of objecting to the parents' demands. The usual answer to any such demands is, "I'm working on that in my therapy!" Treatment may thus serve as an umbrella protecting the adult-child from unwanted parental interventions. Therapy may also furnish the adult-child with a comprehensive catalog of damages, real or presumed, that the parents inflicted on the child. The parents then find out, to their dismay, that the therapy they initiated has become a new source of ammunition in the adult-child's blaming repertoire.

Parents Are Advised to Show Unconditional Acceptance

A common attitude of therapists toward parents is to encourage them to accept their child as is. Adult-children are often believed to suffer from low self-esteem due to past and present failures of parental validation. Although validating a child's experience is certainly important, unconditional acceptance is often interpreted as a big parental hug. Any parental demand is viewed as implicit criticism, which further erodes the adult-child's self-esteem. Not infrequently, the terminology of unconditional acceptance, validation and compensation becomes a guilt trip, justifying endless accommodation. As one of the mothers in our treatment put it, "I allowed my husband to traumatize my daughter and now she's like a chick with broken wings. How can I not take care of her?"

Parents Are Advised to Be Tough

Some professionals understand that so long as parents continue to accommodate the adult-child's expectations, nothing will change. They therefore recommend that parents abruptly cut off all services or even evict the adult-child from the home. When this type of recommendation fails, usually it is because it considers neither the parents' difficulties nor the risks of escalation.

The Decision to Work with the Parents without the Adult-Child's Involvement in Therapy

Parent training is viewed as a valid form of treatment in the case of younger children. However, when the "child" is aged 20 to 30 this may seem odd. Our decision to work with the parents of adult-children was due to the understanding that AED is a systemic problem. Parents are as much part of it as the adult-child. But this would seem to suggest family therapy rather than parent training. In NVR, however, parents (and sometimes other caregivers) are the clients. We do recommend that adult-children receive individual treatment, if they are willing to accept it. However, there are some cogent reasons to view the parents as the main clients.

Parents are Motivated

We believe in the saying that "the client is the one who is ready to sweat!" In AED, parents are almost invariably the willing side. The reason is that they are the ones who shoulder the burden, fear for the future, feel exhausted and are often exploited, blackmailed and victimized.

Parents Deserve Help No Less Than the Adult-Child

Although most parents turn to therapy in order to help their child, and only a few seek help for themselves, their suffering justifies viewing them as clients in their own right. Parental suffering deserves help no less than child suffering. However, it takes considerable persuasion to help parents see things in this light. Parents are so accustomed to meeting their child's needs that they tend to ignore their own. This is characteristic of the dysfunctional bond. Some parents cannot commit to improving their own life until it dawns on them that this is the only way for them to help their child.

Including the Adult-Child in Therapy Distracts the Parents from Doing Their Job

NVR sees the main goals of parents as: (a) reconnecting to their selves, reasserting their own rights, wishes and needs; (b) reasserting their place and influence in the family; (c) resisting aggressive, exploitative and other unacceptable behaviors; and (d) reducing accommodation. The adult-child's presence in therapy usually distracts parents from these goals. Parents of adult-children are so conditioned to place the needs and feelings of their child above their own that the child's emotional reactions in the room would capture all their attention. In addition, adult-children are seldom amenable to the parents' intention to reduce accommodation and in many cases staunchly oppose and try to sabotage it. Planning to de-accommodate is hard enough when the adult-child is absent. Doing so when the adult-child is present can be well-nigh impossible.

Including the Adult-Child in the Therapy Distracts the Therapist from Their Job

NVR therapists are . . . therapists. Their training prepares them to respond with empathy to any emotional need expressed by their clients. In addition, therapists are primed to pay special attention to the suffering of children. The theories that have shaped our thinking as therapists have mostly to do with how parents' faults are visited upon their children, not vice versa. It takes an effort for NVR therapists to relate to parents' needs and suffering, especially as parents often react in problematic ways to their child's difficulties. In such situations, the adult-child's presence in the room would distract the therapist from their hard-won parental focus.

Having said that, NVR therapists do invite the adult-child to one session. A face-to-face meeting with an adult-child helps the therapist assess their condition, improves rapport with the parents, who otherwise may feel uncomfortable "to go behind the child's back," and informs decision making. Many parents ask us how they should invite their children to this session. We offer them the following pitch:

> We realize that we have parenting problems. We are the ones who need help now. We found a therapist who specializes in helping parents. She would like to invite you to one session to see how you can help her help us. We are not trying to trick you into going to therapy. This is a single session. You'd be helping us.

Many adult-children respond positively to this approach, if only because they are eager to tell their side of the story.

This description helps understand why NVR may be especially suited for treating AED, even though some other approaches may seem relevant for many of the adult-children we are describing. For instance, Dialectical Behavior Therapy addresses young adults who are sometimes similar to those whose parents we treat. Dialectical Behavior Therapy includes parents and focuses on escalation by its emphasis on emotional regulation. Moreover, it has proved effective in reducing suicide risk (Ben-Porath, 2010; Harvey et al., 2019). These characteristics might make it relevant for AED. However, we believe there may be a special indication for NVR whenever the adult-child is not willing to cooperate (in Dialectical Behavior Therapy work with the parents is usually an adjunct to work with the child), the parents are exploited or victimized, and there is not only suicide risk, but also specific suicide threats that are raised in a context of intimidation.[1]

The Narrative of Total Responsibility: Past, Present and Future

The parents' desire to convince their child of the need for individual therapy is not a productive undertaking. This desire is emblematic of a more problematic attitude: the belief that the parents are totally responsible for making their child well again. Surely, all parents want their children to be healthy. The problem arises, however, when parents assume responsibility for that outcome. Parents express this kind of problematic responsibility when they ask us: "How can I make her more sociable?" "How can I get him to work?" "How can we make her eat?" "How do I convince him that I don't love his sister more than him?"

Those questions rest on two problematic assumptions. The first is that getting adult-children to do what is good for them is a parental obligation. The second is that the parents have control over this outcome. Let us begin with the second, which we have named the *illusion of control*, that is, parents' belief that they have control over the adult-child's attitudes or behavior (Omer, 2004b; in press). Parents obviously have no control over their child's thoughts and feelings. This applies to young children as well as to adults. Neither do parents have control over children's acts. Parents can occasionally impose their will on a young child, but this behavioral constraint usually vanishes as soon as the child is out of sight. Control is thus an illusion. Parents can only control their own actions.

This brings us back to the first assumption, that parents are obliged to get children to do what is good for them. The illusion of control invalidates the ethical basis of the "narrative of total responsibility," for no one can be held responsible for something over which they have no control. This narrative is also developmentally problematic, since it shifts responsibility away from the child. This is evident both in routine matters as well as in more vital ones. Thus, if a parent constantly reminds a child to do homework or wakes the child up

---

[1] See Chapter 4.

every morning, the child has little chance of assuming those responsibilities; or, if the parent feels totally responsible for the adult-child's financial behavior, the adult-child will probably remain financially irresponsible. Therefore, helping parents liberate themselves from the burden of total responsibility is the first step in freeing the adult-child from being infantilized.

However, the narrative of total responsibility is deeply rooted. Parents often believe they can and should cure their child, not least because they blame themselves for having made the child unwell. Many parents come to us feeling profoundly guilty for having destroyed the life of their child. Even when they blame someone else, usually a spouse, they feel guilty for not having intervened. This sense of guilt over what happened in the past is linked to their feeling of responsibility for what is happening in the present. The parent considers it their absolute duty to take care of the child and compensate for past wrongs. The parent thus becomes the adult-child's oxygen mask. Letting the adult-child down in their precarious moments would be the worst possible betrayal. This sense of responsibility also extends into the future. Many of those parents say to themselves, "Only I can make my child get better." Therefore, the parent must get the child into therapy, bring them to socialize, or arrange for them to find a job. If asked why, the parent will probably answer in dismay, "Who else?"

One goal of NVR is to help parents relinquish both their sense of total responsibility and the illusion of control. Parents can resist or support their children's actions, but they cannot determine them. Therefore, when the parents want to oppose the child's negative behaviors, they should say "*We* will do this." and never "*You* won't do this." In using the first person, the parents are assuming responsibility for their own acts. We also tell parents that we do not think they are the cause of the adult-child's problems. We believe those problems resulted from a convergence of factors, such as genetics, social circumstances, bad influences and bad luck. Perhaps the parents did not know how to prevent the negative outcomes. But how could they have known that their natural protective instincts could have brought about such negative results? Very often the problematic situation has developed despite or because of their loving intentions.

When we succeed in helping parents relinquish those assumptions, the tangles in the parent–child relationship begin to loosen. Degrees of freedom become manifest. Attempts to control the child's fate become less frequent. The parents then become available for the real task at hand: freeing themselves from the dysfunctional bond.

The Effects of Parental Accommodation

The link between accommodation and dysfunction was first shown in the families of children and adults with OCD. Accommodation was shown to be correlated with symptom severity, dysfunction, and with the failure of CBT and medical treatments for the child (Garcia et al., 2010; Storch et al., 2007). It is easy to underestimate the importance of this finding. We are not used to thinking of the success of medical treatment as dependent on an interactional frame. And yet, so long as parental accommodation remains high, medication may fail to have the expected effects. That the same is true of CBT for the child is no less surprising. After all, why should parental accommodation reduce the positive effects of the cognitive and behavior changes fostered by CBT?

The answer is that both medication and CBT can succeed only if they help the child overcome avoidance and confront the feared challenges. However, so long as parental accommodation persists, the child may avoid taking those steps. The parents' protective services actually weaken the child's resolve, undermining the potential positive effects of CBT or medical treatment.

Gradually, research on parental accommodation was extended to a variety of disorders. The effects of accommodation were found to be similar in anxiety disorders, HFASD, eating disorders, dysfunction in the wake of brain concussion, and depression (Shimshoni et al., 2019). An important question was whether helping parents reduce accommodation would improve the child's symptoms and functioning, independently of any other therapy. Some studies have shown this to be the case. The Supportive Parenting for Anxious Childhood Emotions (SPACE) program (Lebowitz & Omer, 2013) is an adaptation of NVR that was designed to help parents of children with anxiety disorders reduce accommodation. The results were promising: Training parents in reducing accommodation led to similar improvements in the child's symptoms and functioning as those achieved by CBT, whether the child agreed or refused to have therapy (Lebowitz et al., 2014; 2020). Interestingly, about 70 percent of the children who had previously refused treatment, agreed to therapy after their parents had completed the training. This was probably due to the fact that they now had nothing to lose, as the parents had already stopped accommodating.

Parents' Difficulties in Stopping Accommodation

Even when parents understand the principle of de-accommodation, they may still object to it. Understanding parental reservations may help therapists overcome these obstacles to change. To improve our dialogue with parents and motivate them to stop accommodating, we must listen attentively and discuss their objections. Here are some arguments therapists should be prepared to hear when working with parents of adult-children:

> *"My child suffers from a mental disability that prevents her from coping."* The belief that the child's problem behavior is due to a mental disorder that poses an insurmountable obstacle to

functioning deters many parents from reducing their accommodation. They feel that doing so would be unfair, like expecting a paraplegic to walk. Parents with this attitude tend to view behavioral problems as rooted in the mind, thus discounting the importance of interpersonal interaction in perpetuating them. Parents of adult-children often fear that, given their child's mental disorder, de-accommodation would be not only unfair but devastating.

"If I stop accommodating, my child will react in dangerous ways." Many parents express the fear that the adult-child would self-harm or harm them in response to de-accommodation. Such fears are perfectly reasonable. Some parents had painful experiences of their child's frightening reactions.

"Only an unloving parent can cause a child such suffering." Those parents believe that de-accommodation would show they did not love their child and that de-accommodating would make them bad parents. Such parents often use their child's suffering as a reason for accommodating. They insist that their accommodation can barely compensate for the child's distress, so de-accommodation would be doubly unfair.

"Life at home will become a battlefield!" Many parents fear that the decision to de-accommodate would start a war of attrition. Even with a young child this fear can be daunting; with an adult-child it can be a veritable horror scenario.

"If I tell others about the problem, my child will feel betrayed." This objection refers to the attempt to mobilize a social support network, which is central to NVR. Such mobilization requires the parents to lift the veil of secrecy surrounding the problem. Many adult-children demand absolute secrecy, sometimes threatening dire consequences, if the parents disclose their problem.

"I simply cannot do it! Every time I tried, I failed!" Many parents feel incapable of de-accommodating since, in the conflict that ensues, the child is stronger than they are. A history of previous defeats convinces those parents they cannot succeed.

Dealing with Parental Objections

Many parents fear that de-accommodation would be traumatically painful to the child. They believe, for instance, that anxiety would rise to the point that the adult-child would collapse. Some of those parents can be helped by some psychoeducation on the self-limiting physiology of anxiety. Normally, when anxiety rises, the body reacts by developing antagonistic responses to the initial elevation of hormones, blood pressure, heart rate and muscle tension that are the physiological underpinnings of fear. The anxiety curve is therefore bell-shaped. Anxiety does not rise indefinitely but goes up and then down. That is why exposure treatments for anxiety are effective. Many parents of anxious children are reassured by this explanation (Lebowitz & Omer, 2013). The same applies to the parents of adult-children. Understanding that the adult-child's condition has been maintained, among other reasons, by their *fear of fear*, helps parents become willing to endure when the adult-child responds with fear (and anger) to their decision to de-accommodate.

A central aspect of this discussion is a reappraisal of the adult-child's endurance. Many parents react positively to the idea that endurance is a capacity that can be cultivated. They often agree that in all probability it would be a blessing for their adult-child to experience situations in which they had no choice but to endure. Parents often ask, "How can we convince our child of the need to endure?" Obviously, telling the adult-child that they can endure is not very helpful, for the adult-child would then try to prove the contrary. This leads to the understanding that the adult-child needs to discover this on their own. Parents cannot simply impart their understandings to the adult-child. They cannot guide and control the adult-child's learning. In fact, most adult-children can only learn that they can endure, when their parents stop their attempts to convince them.

However, the parents can play an active role in this process by cultivating their own capacity to endure. The parent can then tell the child, "In the past I was not so good at enduring situations in which you felt anxious. I now know that I can do so." Thus, instead of telling the adult-child, "I know that you can endure," the parent says, "I know that *I* can endure." In the first case the parent sermonizes, thus provoking the adult-child to prove the parent wrong. In the second, there is no sermon or pep talk. On the contrary, the parents merely reflect on the inner change they have experienced. This is far more convincing, precisely because it involves no attempt to convince.

One central element of NVR that contributes vastly to endurance is support. Gandhi taught that the courage of non-violent resistors is not born in solitude but in togetherness. The experience of support is many-sided. Supporters help parents by giving them a sense of legitimization, by offering to relieve them in some of their tasks, by direct encouragement or simply by staying by their side in difficult moments. Moreover, adult-children tend to behave more maturely in the presence of supporters than when alone with their parents. This happens either because the adult-child is less regressive with those persons or because the mechanism of distress and accommodation is not as closely meshed and well-oiled with supporters as with the parents.

When parents discuss their family problems with supporters in a therapeutic context, they often encounter spontaneous expressions of encouragement and legitimization. Here are some typical examples.

The parents of a 17-year-old girl described in a supporters' meeting that they had not gone out as a couple since their daughter developed an extreme fear of going out or staying alone in the house. The father's brother proposed that, should the parents decide to resume their outings, he would be in touch with the girl by phone, during the first few times. The grandfather, who lived two blocks away, offered to come over for a short visit. This convinced the parents that venturing to go out as a couple was a real possibility. After the parents had gone out a few times on their own, the daughter went out of the house, accompanied by a cousin, for the first time in two years.

The parents of a 14-year-old boy with school refusal and addiction to computer games told the group of their intention to keep the computer turned off during school hours and after 10 o'clock at night. A close family friend who had a good relationship with the boy offered to talk to him about it. She later reported their conversation. When the boy protested against the parents' decision she answered, "Do you want them to give up on you? They can't do that! Neither can I!"

Parental endurance is boosted when parents are relieved, even if temporarily, from their total involvement with the adult-child. In NVR training we explore how the less involved parent can relieve the other in difficult situations. Grandparents may also be well-suited for these tasks, especially if they are not major suppliers of accommodation services. Whoever the supporters are, it is important to brief them on the damages of accommodation, in order to help them better withstand the child's pressure. This kind of support alleviates the parents' fear of being perceived as "bad parents."

However, many parents are reluctant to ask others for help. The usual parental reservations are: (a) they fear this would expose them as weak; (b) they believe that revealing the secret would cause the child unbearable shame; (c) they feel that no supporters are available; and (d) they fear the child might react in extreme ways. We have developed several ways of dealing with those reservations.

Parents who fear that asking for support exposes them as weak are helped to view support as empowering. Far from making them appear weak, support lends them a new kind of strength, that of saying "We" instead of "I." This transition to the first person plural is central to NVR. The child often taunts the parents for running to others for help. The parents learn to reply proudly, "Our only mistake was staying alone for so long."

Regarding shame, parents are helped by the consideration that there are negative and positive kinds of shame. Negative shame is the shame of exclusion (e.g., "You don't belong here."), which is the opposite of what happens when shame is experienced in a supportive context. Supporters are specifically instructed to create a positive context by expressing their care and appreciation, by telling the adult-child they believe they can overcome the difficulty and by offering to help the adult-child find a solution. Many parents connect well to the idea of "constructive shame," and that by keeping things secret the child is actually deprived of this vital experience.

Parents who say they have no available supporters can be encouraged to proactively examine that assumption. Many parents reduce social contact with friends or extended family out of shame about their child's condition. Reversing this self-imposed seclusion can be a turning point. Sometimes, parents rule out certain types of supporters – such as grandparents – arguing they should not be bothered, either because of their age and health condition, or because they are preoccupied with their own problems. Most parents can be convinced that excluding grandparents is probably a bad way of being considerate. In effect, the reaction of grandparents to parents' request for help is almost invariably supportive, showing not only a willingness to cooperate, but also that helping their child (the parent) and grandchild is deeply meaningful to them. Therapists who take the trouble to explore parents' reservations often succeed in convincing them to build a significant support group. It turns out that this is a learnable skill. Experienced therapists in our center can be quite successful in motivating parents to create a support network.

The chief difficulty that parents have, both in terms of the involvement of supporters and the entire project of de-accommodation, is fear of the adult-child's overreaction. In NVR training, those fears are never dismissed. On the contrary, they are given serious consideration and the parents are helped to develop appropriate coping strategies.

One of the frightening issues that NVR training always covers is the fear of escalation. Parents are helped to understand both *symmetrical* and *complementary* escalation. In symmetrical escalation, parents and child have similar reactions (blaming, yelling at and threatening each other), with each response intensifying the cycle. In complementary escalation, concessions from the parents only make the adult-child more demanding.

A particularly nefarious complementary dynamic is blackmail; when parents give in to the adult-child, the adult-child is emboldened to pressure them even more. In NVR training, parents learn to identify and avoid both kinds of escalation. Training in NVR helps parents to see where they are vulnerable and what triggers them. They role-play to prepare for explosive situations, learn to delay their reactions, refrain from domineering messages and convey respectful determination. Supporters can also be very helpful in reducing the risk of escalation. Thus, when supporters are present, there is almost always less violence. Parents are encouraged to call their supporters when they suspect a potentially explosive situation. Their mere presence, sometimes even by phone, offers protection to the parents and helps defuse the situation. They can also mediate, helping bring the parents and adult-child to an acceptable compromise. Supporters can also invite the adult-child to spend time with them, giving both the child and parents a respite. The time adult-children spend away from home often reveals their more functional side.

An important part in NVR training, which answers many objections that parents might have, is a careful preparation for worst-case scenarios. These scenarios provide a fuzzy background to the parents' accommodation. Sometimes, simply discussing those scenarios is empowering for parents. A typical example is the fear that the adult-child will react to the parents' steps by moving out, adopting a high-risk lifestyle or becoming homeless. The reason this kind of script often dissipates in the telling is that it contradicts all that the parents know about their child. For instance, a fastidious, control-obsessed and territorial young person is hardly likely to sleep under a bridge. Similarly, a deeply anxious and withdrawn adolescent will hardly become a delinquent. Parents can be guided to understand that their adult-child would not get into the type of trouble that is totally uncharacteristic of them. It is useful for many parents to visualize the real developmental threats facing their child. For instance, "The biggest threat to your child is that of becoming completely isolated." or "His foremost risk is abandoning the real world in favor of the virtual world." In saying those things, the therapist is not showing a gift of prophecy but merely extrapolating from what is happening in the present to what will probably happen in the future.

The most useful narratives for helping parents deal with their own frightening scenarios include not only what the adult-child might do, but also what the parents could do. Detailed scripts can be prepared, including the parent's de-accommodation steps, the probable reactions by the adult-child, and the parents' preparation to cope with those reactions. Parents can learn how best to react to a variety of situations such as being threatened or physically attacked, property being destroyed, the adult-child going missing or screaming in the middle of the night. Making detailed plans to face these eventualities is an essential part of NVR training.

The most unthinkable scenario for parents is that of the adult-child's suicide. Surprisingly, although there is an abundance of professional articles on suicidality, there is virtually no research on how to cope when the child utters suicide threats. And yet, this is a common phenomenon, which causes enormous suffering to parents and sometimes jeopardizes the entire de-accommodation project. As this is a central fear for many parents, we have devoted a special chapter to it.[2]

Listening patiently to parents' objections is a crucial element in the creation of a positive and stable therapeutic alliance. Whenever parents say that they are struggling with a therapeutic step, the therapist should pay close attention. Parents' apparent lack of cooperation should not be attributed to a lack of

---

[2] Chapter 4.

motivation but rather to real dilemmas that need attention. The important questions for the therapist to ask in those circumstances are, "What is making this step difficult for you?" "Can you think of any modifications that might make it easier?" "What additional help do you think you need?" When the therapist considers these issues openly and with care, many parents who had previously been unable to act, feel empowered to do so.

Treatment Goals

Parents often ask us about our success rate. This question requires us to clarify our goals and our definition of success. A realistic notion of what can and cannot be achieved is crucial for maintaining a good working alliance, and for keeping parents motivated and prepared.

The chief goal of treatment, as already mentioned, is the gradual transformation of dysfunctional into functional dependence. As parents are the direct clients of the intervention, we expect change to manifest first with them. When parents ask, "But what about my child, will he get better?" "Will she marry, work, be independent?," it is important to reiterate, "You don't have any control over your child, but you can gain better control over yourselves. By improving your side of the problem, you provide your child with far better chances of improvement."

NVR improves the readiness and ability of parents to stop accommodating by helping them develop a number of crucial competences, such as: confronting their own catastrophic scenarios; reducing escalation; overcoming helplessness; amassing support; cooperating better as a couple; defending themselves against violence, humiliation and exploitation; enriching their repertoire of effective reactions; and attending to their own well-being. At the risk of being repetitive, we want to stress that the parents' suffering is no less deserving of attention than their child's. Moreover, unless parents become willing to help themselves, they will not be able to help their child.

Improvements in the parents are usually followed by improvements in the adult-child, such as: violence diminishes; anxiety and depression lift; social relations improve; self-isolation and computer addiction wane; and many begin (or resume) working or studying (Lebowitz et al., 2012).

Some goals, which are important to many parents, are not suitable for NVR. The therapist should make this clear to the parents whenever they raise the issue. Among these goals are getting the adult-child to go to therapy; convincing the adult-child to take medication; curing the adult-child's underlying disorder; and making the adult-child happy. These goals are not acceptable because, by insisting on them, parents reduce the chances that they may be achieved. As we said before, parents cannot make those things happen. All they can do is create the conditions that make them possible.

3   The Intervention

We have described entrenched dependence as a co-constructed reality in which the parent and the adult-child become bonded and at the same time isolated from their social world. The intervention starts by helping parents relinquish their narrative of total responsibility for the adult-child's condition and focus on self-change. This chapter introduces steps and tools for helping parents give up this narrative; shift their focus to themselves; garner support; resist their adult-child's pressure, threats and violence; de-accommodate to dysfunctional expectations; and cope with their own fears in constructive ways.

De-accommodation may risk confrontation and escalation. A major intervention challenge facing the therapist is to minimize this risk, while allowing parents to preserve and cultivate the best parts of their relationship with the adult-child. NVR is suited for this challenge, as an approach of constructive struggle (Alon & Omer, 2006) that aims to reduce conflict and promote mutual healing.

Settings and Course

Clients

The intervention is conducted with one or both parents or primary caregivers. The process applies to adult-children as well as adolescents manifesting dysfunctional dependence patterns similar to those we have described. Parents usually initiate the intervention, but sometimes other family members do it for them, in which case these family members attend the first session. The adult-child attends only one individual session with the therapist, if they accept the invitation to come.

Intervention Duration and Pace

Interventions usually consist of 10 to 20 sessions. The first sessions are held weekly but may become less frequent as the parents acquire coping skills. One session, usually longer, is held with the family's support network. Occasionally the treatment process is put on standby, when there has been some progress (for instance, when the situation at home stabilizes and the adult-child starts functioning better), and parents are advised to return in case of relapse. During an acute crisis, there might be two or even three sessions during the same week.

Diagnoses

The intervention is neither indicated nor counter-indicated by any psychiatric diagnosis. We have applied it with parents of adult-children on a diagnostic range that spans OCD, social phobia, Post-Traumatic Stress Disorder (PTSD), ADHD, HFASD, learning disabilities, bipolar disorder, schizophrenia, personality disorder, panic disorder, eating disorder or without any diagnosis. The great majority of the adult-children involved in our cases were not in employment, school or training. Most of them lived in the parental home. Those who did not were invariably supported by their parents, financially and otherwise. The only common denominator across the diagnostic range was a rigid, dysfunctional dependence in which the parents performed extensive and age-inappropriate services for the adult-child. In treating AED, we are addressing the dysfunctional bond that plays a major role in perpetuating the problem and distress on both sides. The adult-child may or may not be in treatment for their underlying disorder. When they are, we aim at establishing a collaborative dialogue with the professionals in charge of the adult-child's treatment.

Age Range

The children whose parents we saw ranged in age from 16 to 45. In adolescents, this treatment is especially indicated when high dysfunction is coupled with a dependence bond. Among these are adolescents who refuse to attend school, misuse the Internet, sever their social ties, shut themselves up in their rooms or force parents to comply with their dysfunctional demands.

Teamwork

Because of the complexity and high threat potential of those cases, it is highly recommended that therapy be conducted in team settings, whether in an established clinic or a mutual help professional group. However, parent counselors can use this manual on their own for purposes of prevention in lighter cases with worrying signs but not a chronic picture of entrenched dependence.[1]

---

[1] See Chapter 5.

Intervention Course

Although the intervention's course and length may vary greatly between families, it does follow a characteristic arc that can serve as a roadmap. Describing this arc to the parents is in itself therapeutic, as it provides them with a time perspective and prepares them for the challenges ahead. At the opening stage, the therapist and parents develop a picture of the dysfunctional bond; of the adult-child's difficulties and strengths; and of the trajectory that led the parents and the adult-child to their present condition. The therapist then introduces the goals of treatment: protect themselves from pressures, attacks and exploitation, reduce accommodation and prevent escalation.

The second stage is characterized by two parallel processes: preparing and delivering a formal announcement to the adult-child, in which the parents declare the changes they will undertake and the behaviors they will resist; and recruiting a supportive network of relatives and friends.

The third stage comprises the actual work of de-accommodation. Parents gradually stop catering to their adult-child and find nonescalating ways of coping with the adult-child's adverse reactions. The intervention concludes with a review of what has been accomplished and thoughts preparing the parents for possible future difficulties. Some parents return at a later time for a few sessions to get assistance with a crisis or threat of relapse.

The Opening Stage

The opening stage usually spans three to four sessions and comprises the following tasks.

Establishing a Working Alliance

The primary objective of the opening stage is to offer parents a space of their own, where they can consider their own wellness, needs, interests and goals and find better ways of coping with their adult-child. To many parents, it is not at all obvious that they are not only the therapy's instruments but also its clients. When parents come to us, they are usually too effaced as individuals and so immersed in their child's problems that they cannot see themselves as anything but conduits to the child's wellness. The therapist's task is to help them distance themselves from the maelstrom of pressures and provocations. By viewing them both as parents and as persons in their own right, the therapist creates a safe distance away from the stifling immediacy of their "home planet," enabling an observable "there." From this vantage point, parents discover that they can be proactive instead of reactive. They then begin planning and implementing new ways of acting and living.

The therapeutic attitude conveys the feeling that the therapist is on the parents' side, understands their pain and respects their wishes and efforts; promotes a shared goal that is attractive to and acceptable for the parents; and helps them acquire the means to reach that goal, while paying close attention to their concerns. At the conclusion of the opening stage, parents should have a clear idea of the work ahead, a sense of renewed possibility and a sense that the therapist they chose can guide and assist them in carrying out that work.

Developing a Picture of the Problem that Allows for New Options

In every life domain that parents describe, the therapist seeks to identify exceptions or signs of flexibility that may counter the parents' pessimistic outlook. However, the therapist should not minimize their difficulties. Rushing to solutions may offend the parents and harm the chances for a good working alliance. It is important to keep focused on the present, for the tendency to delve into the adult-child's past may stifle hope. Therefore, parents are asked to begin by describing their difficulties at *present*. If they wish to start with the past and explain how the present situation developed, the therapist may say, "We will do that soon, but first I would like to hear a brief description of the present difficulties, so that I can better understand how they developed." An adequate picture of the present situation should include *the adult-child's daily routine* (e.g., sleeping and waking cycle, occupations and preoccupations, and interpersonal relations), *problematic behaviors* (e.g., verbal or physical violence, self-harmful or suicidal acts or threats, and compulsive behaviors), *areas of functioning* (e.g., work, study, driving, helping others and interest areas) and *relationship with the parents and others*. As parents describe each of these elements, the therapist asks for how long these patterns have been manifest and whether there were times when the adult-child behaved differently.

When a positive event is identified, the therapist may say, "This shows she can function better in this respect" or "We see he has abilities that fluctuate according to circumstances." Parents usually respond well to this kind of comment, especially if the therapist takes care not to underrate their difficulties. For instance, the therapist may say, "Considering that he is capable of that, I can imagine how frustrating it is that he usually doesn't do it."

Parents are then asked to describe how the adult-child developed; when the first signs of the problem appeared; the adult-child's academic and occupational history; best life periods; achievements and reactions to failure; and how the parents had coped with difficulties in the past. It is important to focus on turning points. Times of improved functioning, even if temporary, tell us something about the circumstances that may have enabled them. Negative turning points indicate potential obstacles. Turning points may show that dysfunctional dependence is not an immutable condition. This can raise hope and motivation for change. Motivation, in contrast, can also be stimulated by considering the static side of dysfunctional dependence. Thus, the therapist may inquire how long difficult periods have lasted in the adult-child's life. When parents begin dating the process and accounting for all the years that have passed with no change, except their getting older, they may be shocked into a higher readiness for action.

In the biography of adult-children, there are almost always periods of better functioning. Many parents tell of the adult-child's success with studies, employment, times in which the adult-child lived outside the parental home, friendships, intimate relationships or trips abroad. The significance of these events is often lost under the massive weight of the present dysfunction. It takes an active effort to look at them closely and salvage the valuable information they contain about the adult-child's functioning potential.

In cases of entrenched dependence, virtually all those positive attempts eventually collapse. Academic studies are discontinued, relationships break down and work is interrupted. The therapist asks the parents to describe what, to their minds, led the adult-child to give up and how they reacted. These negative turning points arouse the protective instincts of almost any caring parent. However, whereas in other families, young persons may eventually get back on their feet, in adult-children this fails to happen. Rather, demoralization and dependence deepen and parents settle into their protective role.

Discussing Parental Accommodation

After the parents elaborate the family's present condition and the problem's history, it is a good time to discuss *accommodation*. Most parents grasp that the services they perform for the adult-child are inadequate. The therapist should strengthen this understanding by explaining how accommodation only deepens dysfunction and leads to greater anxiety and withdrawal. Most parents understand how, in their attempt to rescue their adult-child, they may achieve the opposite. It is important to listen empathically to the parents' explanation why they cannot simply stop performing the services that the adult-child has come to expect. The therapist agrees with the parents that they cannot abruptly terminate their services, however inadequate and damaging. The therapist's job is to help them do that in a gradual, safe and constructive way.

This conversation can recur many times during sessions. In discussing the innumerable ways in which accommodation is manifested, the therapist aims to untangle the family's mesh of protectiveness and distress. We nicknamed this process "therapeutic plowing," as it consists in burrowing into the patterns that prevent any slackening of parental services, so that the seeds of change may take root.

A helpful image for the damages of accommodation is that of the parental home as a *degenerative shelter*, or a *den of stagnation*, that instead of allowing the adult-child to get better, fosters decay. The goal of therapy is to dismantle that shelter.

Addressing the Assumption of Total Responsibility

It is crucial to stress to the parents that stopping accommodation will not immediately bring the adult-child to function, but rather create the conditions that make it possible. This clarification often raises parental questions like, "But how can we convince him that this is for his good?" "How do we bring her out of the protective shelter and into the world?" "How do we get him to work?" These questions reflect the narrative of total responsibility. The therapist should patiently explain that the more the parents try to force these outcomes, the more the adult-child will resist. The parents will repeatedly ask, "But eventually will he function?" Repeatedly, the therapist should answer, "When you stop accommodating, you provide your child a real chance of functioning and living better. But you have no direct control over that. It is not you who can bring him to work, study and socialize."

Although parents may understand this in principle, the narrative of total responsibility needs repeated attention as they take practical steps along the intervention's arc. The more parents become empowered to act, the better they understand, and vice versa.

Discussing the Need for a Support Network

The lack of a social support network is closely related to the establishment of a degenerative shelter. Parental isolation is both an effect and a cause of degeneration. An effect, because parents often reduce contact with their surroundings out of shame for what is happening at home or because of the adult-child's absolute demands for secrecy. A cause, since the more isolated the family, the harder it becomes to expose it to positive inputs and options. A closed family system avoids stimuli. The more isolated the family, the more hopeless the situation. The process of gathering support is both daunting and inspiring. It is daunting because parents have to overcome their shame and fear. It is inspiring because the help and solidarity conveyed by the support group strengthens the parents and opens windows to the world. A therapist may bring up the idea of a support network, by connecting it to the metaphor of the degenerative shelter:

I do not expect you to go home after this meeting and dismantle the degenerative shelter that you have unwittingly come to provide your child. You will need help in order to do that. Parents who try to cope alone with this complex task are too weak and vulnerable to do it well. Your child knows all too well how to push your buttons. The situation changes completely once you are surrounded by relatives and close friends. I imagine that the thought of involving other people in what is happening in your home may not be easy. We can discuss this difficulty later and explore ways to deal with any concerns you may have. But I want you to know that, once you have rallied support, your life and the life of your child will no longer be the same.

Learning How to Prevent Escalation

NVR is by definition not only strictly non-violent but also nonescalating. NVR practitioners, both in the socio-political and in the family field, carefully avoid provocation or retaliation. Escalation is a major factor in perpetuating parental accommodation, because parents become scared when their attempts at change lead to harsh confrontations. Helping parents understand the dynamics of escalation and providing them tools to diminish their own contribution to those processes is an important task to be addressed from the outset. The following principles and skills, which we have used in NVR training for many different conditions, have been demonstrated to achieve those goals (Omer, 2004b).

> *"Strike while the iron is cold."* This flip side of the saying, "strike while the iron is hot," is geared to helping parents resist the temptation to react immediately to an adult-child's acts and provocations. It reduces escalation by allowing parents to cool down before responding or helping them rein in their impulse to rush to the adult-child's rescue at the first sign of distress. Most parents can understand that the goal of the adult-child's provocations is to spark an angry or protective reaction. Whenever they react like that, parents are actually "falling into the trap." Understanding this, they can develop the ability to say, "We do not accept that. We will consider our steps and notify you later." There are many gains in delaying their reaction: the atmosphere becomes calmer, the parents build up resilience and the tight action–reaction patterns that maintain the dependence bond are loosened.

> *"You do not have to win but only to persist."* One of the harmful causes of escalation is the belief that problems can be resolved by a show of force. This attitude is highly destructive, because it may lead to ever stronger blows. This problematic stance is illustrated by the ironic saying: "What cannot be achieved by force – can be achieved by more force." This attitude turns the relationship between parent and child into a sequence of showdowns, each of which not only fails to achieve either side's goal, but guarantees that each confrontation will be worse than the last. The belief in sheer force leads to

extreme reactions that alternate with parental giving in. In contrast, the maxim, "You do not have to win but only to persist," is based on the assumption that improvements will ripen, if the parents persevere. The required persistence is not a rigid repetition of the same actions but is expressed by the willingness to continue seeking solutions, patiently striving for partial improvements and developing sensitivity to the slightest signs of positive change.

"I have no control over you but only over me." The parents' attempts to control the adult-child almost invariably backfire. However, standing firm is not the same as trying to control. When parents present a firm stance, they are exercising control over themselves, not over their child. The parent is not saying to the adult-child, "You will do what I say!" but rather, "I will do what I say!" Giving up the illusion of control and focusing on self-control is hard for many parents. They may say, "So, when she curses me, am I supposed to just sit there?" "Am I supposed to let him walk all over me?"

We do not disregard the question of power but address it openly. We say, "You must be much stronger than you are today, but strong in a different way." The best metaphor for parental firmness is the anchor: "When your child attacks you, you don't strike back, but stay firm like an anchor."

"Identify and avoid 'ping-pong' interactions." Escalation is often marked by rigid symmetrical interchanges guided by a tit-for-tat mentality. Parents show this tendency when they repeatedly ask, "What do I say when she says … [so and so]?" Or "If so and so happens, how do I answer?" The best answer is usually "Nothing!" Learning to break free from the compulsion to answer is an important step toward breaking the grip of escalation on the relationship.

"Don't preach, argue or attempt to convince." When parents try to persuade, they usually lead the adult-child to react sharply or double down. Many parents insist that the adult-child should go to therapy, begin socializing or find a job. Each persuasion attempt is another turn of the screw. Avoiding these counterproductive persuasion attempts can have a de-escalating effect. It may be a good idea to tell the adult-child, "I understand that my nagging is disrespectful and counterproductive. I'll do my best to stop it. If I fall back into it, please remind me."

"Use supporters to defuse explosive situations." Parents are sometimes afraid of bringing in supporters, perhaps fearing an outburst from the adult-child. This occasionally happens, especially the first time that the adult-child is exposed to supporters. Afterwards, their effect on escalation becomes invariably positive. Calling a

supporter usually has a calming effect on the adult-child. The presence of a supporter is probably the best deterrent against physical violence. Supporters also help mediate and achieve compromises. They can also invite the adult-child to go out or spend some time with them, deflecting an escalation.

Providing a Roadmap for the Therapeutic Process

Giving parents an overview of the treatment plan conveys a sense of security. The following text illustrates how this can be done:

I want to describe to you what will be our next steps. We will begin by learning what the problematic services and accommodating acts are by which you unwittingly enable your child's dysfunctional dependence. We will learn to identify the pitfalls that lead to escalation between you and develop ways to avoid them. We will develop a joint plan for dismantling the degenerative shelter and replacing overprotection with positive support. We shall then prepare an announcement, which is a semi-formal declaration by which you notify your child about the changes you are going to undertake. The announcement is delivered both in written form and by word of mouth. This formality is intended to connote a rite of passage, signaling the beginning of a new stage in the life of your family. I will help you prepare for delivering the announcement and cope with your child's response to it. Concurrently, we will discuss how to rally support and what you can reasonably expect from your supporters. If you have any reservations about this process, I will be happy to discuss them with you. We will do one longer session together with your supporters (about 90 to 120 minutes). The introduction of supporters changes the ecology of the problem. Your child will not participate in this gathering. But they would know, by and by, that you are no longer alone and keeping the problems secret. After the supporters' gathering, a mailing list of all supporters will be compiled and they will be regularly notified of new developments. After the announcement and the supporters' session, we will initiate a gradual and systematic process of de-accommodation. We will help you prepare yourselves to cope with your child's reactions, so that you may withstand them without giving in or lashing back. We will seriously consider ways of protecting you and your child from those reactions. The process of de-accommodation will open new options for you and your child. We will be on the lookout for any positive signs of change, as these are sometimes difficult to notice. It is important to resist the temptation to "push the river," that is, to try and get your child to do the things you would wish them to do. All you can do is stop doing the things that keep the situation stuck and offer support in the direction your child may choose to go. Our goal is not the ambitious one of rendering your child fully independent but changing your relationship from one of dysfunctional to one of functional dependence. But that would make all the difference.

This roadmap is a source of hope. Its goals are not total, immediate or unrealistic. Given the great amount of preparation and support involved, the project may seem accessible and the tasks manageable. We know that parents find this vision, which is common to all NVR programs, eminently acceptable.

For this reason, we recommend that the therapist provide the parents a written version of the therapy plan. Each therapist may modify this example, to suit their own style.

Addressing Some Typical Questions

Parents often ask three questions toward the end of the opening session:
1. "Should we tell our child we are in therapy?"
2. "Will the treatment include our child?"
3. "What do we do now?"

We encourage parents to tell their child that they are in therapy. There are three reasons for that. First, transparency is a central value in NVR and by honestly telling their child they have decided to get professional help for themselves, the parents display a new openness that often contrasts with previous secrecy. Second, parents sometimes avoid telling the adult-child they are getting help out of fear for their reactions ("How dare you talk about me to another person behind my back?"). Fear engenders fear, so by not informing the child, parents are giving in to a negative emotion that reinforces the status quo. Third, the child's reaction almost always includes hope and not just protest. Although adult-children seem vested in perpetuating parental services, they also deeply yearn for their condition to change. We tell parents that these unspoken wishes constitute "the change party" within the adult-child's "inner parliament." We assume that in this inner parliament there are always positive voices. However, given the parents' continuous accommodation, those voices are silenced. The situation changes when parents stop accommodating, learn to avoid escalation and mobilize support.

Regarding the second question, we encourage parents to invite the adult-child to a single individual session with the therapist. Parents are briefed to say to their child,

> You have told us numerous times in the past that if there is a problem, it's ours and not yours, and that we should seek help. We realized that this is true, and we are currently seeing a therapist who is helping us with our problem. The therapist thinks that meeting you once would help her to help us with our problem.

Many adult-children respond well to this proposal. Parents also feel helped by the fact that the therapist has met with their child and now has a first-hand impression of the child's difficulties. It is important that the therapist does not attempt to convince the adult-child that the parents' therapy is good for her. If the adult-child expresses a desire for therapy, she will be referred to another therapist.

We strongly recommend that the therapist does not take the adult-child as a client, in parallel to working with the parents. Such a setting would create unnecessary complications and conflicts of loyalty. If the adult-child accepts the offer to go to therapy (or is already in therapy), it is worthwhile to develop a collaborative relationship with the adult-child's therapist, as it can greatly benefit work with the parents. Sometimes, however, the adult-child does not authorize their therapist to release any information to the parents' therapist. In cases like these, most therapists agree to receive authorized updates from the parents' therapist, as this can't infringe their client's confidentiality. We shall elaborate on this point in Chapters 6 and 7.

The third question, "What do we do now?," stems from parents' sometimes shocked understanding that their approach to the adult-child is probably harmful. Even though they can't be expected to change it after one or two sessions, they can still take some initial steps in that direction. One such step is to begin keeping a journal of their interactions with their child. This journal brings to light many automatic acts of accommodation as well as some of the typical escalatory interchanges between them and the adult-child. Parents are encouraged to devote special attention to any demeaning or exploitative moments in the interaction. This new awareness tends to change the way in which parents usually react. It is difficult for the parents to continue a pattern that they now see as humiliating and exploitative. These initial changes are grist to the therapeutic mill and help prepare the parents for the more significant steps that will follow.

The Announcement

An announcement is akin to a rite of passage: a festive, formal and socially validated event that marks a transition of status. Some rites of passage are a confirmation, bar mitzvah, marriage, divorce, signing a contract or graduation. In all of these examples, the change of status is marked by a special event attended not only by the people directly involved but also by witnesses who confirm and validate it. The reason for the formal atmosphere and involvement of others is the need to draw a boundary that enables participants to think, feel and act differently.

The announcement parents are asked to prepare for their adult-children is intended to signal their transition away from accommodation and passivity. Delivering the announcement is thus the formal opening act of the parental resistance campaign. The announcement is not a contract but a declaration: "Here we stand. This is how we have decided to conduct our lives." The preparation for the announcement is no less crucial than its delivery. In developing their announcement, parents internalize its principles, coordinate their positions, summon up the courage to deliver it and prepare to cope with the adult-child's reaction.

Some parents are uncomfortable making a formal announcement, preferring a more natural and spontaneous conversation. The point, however, is precisely to mark a transition in a way that makes it other than "natural," especially as what the parents see as natural, or spontaneous, is a pattern of stagnation, violence, fear and despair. When the announcement is delivered both orally and in writing in a quasi-formal way, it codifies the parents' decision to change. Parents who do this convey the message: "This is a special occasion."

The announcement itself is a concise but comprehensive description of two or three areas in which the parents' behavior will change. For instance, "We shall resist violence and intimidation"; "We shall no longer provide you with services that are not appropriate for someone your age"; "We will no longer come to your rescue when you get into financial trouble"; or "We will no longer obey your commands or abide by your rules regarding meals, hygiene, order, money, noise, social contact or other impositions."

Sometimes, the announcement includes a highly specific item, like, "We will not agree that the computer or TV are on at night in our house" or "We will gradually terminate your monthly allowance over four months." Such items lend the announcement a highly pragmatic tone. It is important, however, that the announcement does not become a long list of services to be withheld. Only two or three areas of resistance should be specifically mentioned, so as not to dilute the parents' message.

If parents raise the concern that many harmful behaviors are not covered by the announcement, it is important to explain that the scope of change they are undertaking goes far beyond what the announcement specifies. The announcement is not an exhaustive list but an opening act. Some parents mention their own limitations (for instance, their age or financial situation) in their announcement or their right to live a fuller life. These are valuable personal additions that give the announcement a deeper human tone. One element that should always figure in the announcement is the parents' decision to lift the veil of secrecy and obtain support wherever they can find it.

Parents vary on the length and prolixity of the announcement, some preferring to be as succinct as possible. One widower, who had been extorted by his 30-year-old gambling-addicted son, delivered the shortest possible announcement: "No more!" After discussing other versions, the therapist and the father reached the conclusion that this message would do the job better than any other.

The announcement is always written in the first person plural ("We"). It is never stated as a prohibition, such as "You must not scream at us or threaten us." The reason is twofold: the language of prohibition invites the adult-child to prove the parents wrong and the prohibition reduces personal presence. Commands sound impersonal; impersonality is exactly what we want to avoid.

The announcement is a unilateral message in which the parents declare a change in their attitude. The adult-child is not asked to comply, since nothing is demanded of them. Neither is the child asked to agree, since nothing is proposed to them. Parents often say, "But she will never agree!" These parents believe that any position they take is meaningless unless their child agrees to it. The announcement signals a change in this very belief. Even if the adult-child protests, resists or ignores it; or crumples up the page; or walks out immediately after it begins, the announcement cannot be annulled (one combative adolescent went so far as to eat the page). On the contrary, the adult-child's reaction allows the parents to say, "You're not expected to agree. We are telling you what *we* are going to do. We gave you a copy of our announcement out of fairness, so as not to act behind your back."

Many parents find it difficult to make a clear announcement. For them, a statement that conveyed unshaken parental resolve would feel like a violation of a sacred taboo. Many of them feel the need to soften their statement with justifications, explanations and apologies. When they set out to demand something, they quickly go from request to apology. The announcement enables a clear stand against the drift.

Some parents fear that the announcement will trigger an extreme response by the adult-child. In such cases, it is recommended to wait with the delivery of the announcement until after the supporters' gathering is convened. Other parents prefer to immediately proceed with the announcement and not wait for their supporters to gather. They should be encouraged, but the therapist should verify that they are prepared to contain the possible escalation that the announcement might trigger and that they have not given up on the idea of getting support.

Parents are encouraged to explore various scenarios of the adult-child's reaction to the announcement and how they might cope in each case. Therapists who use role-playing in their work might invite parents to stage the scene. Many parents show humor and creativity, as they take turns playing the role of their child. The enacted adult-child screams, covers their ears, makes noises, snatches the announcement from the parent's hands, lies down on the couch with their face to the wall, bursts into tears or begs the parents to relent. The role-playing parent's mission is to resist these disruptions by continuing to read from the page. If this reading becomes physically impossible, the parent can conclude the delivery by saying, "We did not expect you to listen to what we have to say. But we are going to do exactly as we write here. We will post a copy on the refrigerator. You may read it if you like. Whether you do or not, we will proceed." If the adult-child makes it impossible for the parents even to say this, they can slip a note to that effect under the child's door later that day. This preparation makes many parents feel that, perhaps for the first time in years, they are acting in a way that is independent of their child's reaction.

Preparing the announcement helps parents address most of their concerns about the risks and consequences of de-accommodation. Parents, who as a result of this preparation have become more capable of dealing with the adult-child's reactions to the announcement, are rapidly advancing toward the ability to de-accommodate. Therefore, dedicating two or even three sessions to preparing the announcement is not wasted time. It encourages and strengthens them for the challenges ahead.

Here is text of an announcement delivered to a 28 year old, who used to live on his own and completed a bachelor's degree in History. He then returned to the parental home, isolated himself, stopped communicating with his parents and spent all of his time on the computer.

Dear Gene,

We have decided to turn to therapy for help on our problems with you. Here is some background we'd like to share with you.

We are now 66 and 62 years old and feel a need to make some essential changes in our lives. For the past four years, since you returned to live at our home, we feel we have developed the wrong habits and attitudes.

We know you are strong-willed and that, no matter what our wishes, we cannot control your choices and behaviors. We cannot convince you that you have a problem or that you need therapy. We cannot get you to leave your room or find a job. We know that you will do exactly what you want. However, we have our own desires and plans. And we've decided that we'll not allow you to determine the way we live our lives and manage our home.

Therefore, we would like to announce to you our major decisions:

We'll no longer provide you with services that are inappropriate for your age and ours. We'll no longer cook for you, wash for you, clean your room, pay for your needs or provide you with Internet.

We have decided not to support a lifestyle in which night and day are reversed. We will therefore take steps to shut down the television and personal computers at home between 23:00 and 8:00. These are our home and our resources, and we will resist what we see as their inappropriate use.

We are sharing with you that we have notified all those who are close to us about our decision. We have asked them to support us. It was not easy for us to overcome our habit of keeping things secret, but we understood that real change requires disclosure. Our house, which has been long closed to visitors, will from now on be open to them.

We trust your ability to make something of your life. We think that by collaborating with your seclusion, we have actually demonstrated lack of trust. We think that was deeply wrong, both for us as parents and for you as the loved and valued son that you are.

Your loving parents

Support

Preparing the announcement makes many parents feel ready to act. Some are willing to proceed with the announcement, while others prefer to wait until they are backed by a support group. If parents prefer to deliver the announcement without having met with their supporters, this is no excuse for avoiding or postponing the supporters' meeting. That could jeopardize the entire intervention, as social support is a critical factor in its success.

Families with dysfunctional dependence often suffer from social isolation. In many cases parents cut off nearly all contact with relatives and friends. Some of the parents we saw reported that difficulties at home and their sense of total responsibility were compromising their performance at work. Some of them even went into early retirement, so as to dedicate themselves fully to the needs of their child. Sometimes, the decision to retire was already taken during the adult-child's adolescence. We think that such decisions tend to exacerbate dysfunctional dependence. Another aggravating factor is when siblings of adult-children, who have already left the parental home, avoid visiting their parents because of its oppressive atmosphere. Life in such families is epitomized by the fact that the shutters are closed.

In less extreme cases, parents maintain their social contacts, allowing others a glimpse into the family's condition. However, the "hard core" events from which they suffer, such as violence, blackmail and suicide threats, are almost always kept secret. The digital culture, compartmentalized urban environment and shrinking of the extended family tend to worsen the family's isolation.

Most parents who come to us attribute their isolation to their adult-child's problematic behaviors. They hide because they are ashamed. This explanation is valid, but the causal link goes both ways. Isolation is both a result and a cause of the dysfunction. Rallying a support network is thus a major step forward.

A support network gives parents the strength and legitimization they need to break free of oppressive patterns. There is little chance that they would overcome their fear and despair without support, hence the considerable efforts we as therapists invest in persuading them to rally sufficient support.

Persuading Parents to Gather Support

Parents are asked to share their difficulties and the fact that they are in therapy with a group of close relatives and friends. They invite their supporters to attend a joint therapy session, and learn more about the family's condition and the effort to change it, as well as discuss possible ways of assisting their efforts. The group would customarily include members of the extended family, the adult-child's adult siblings, parents' close friends and colleagues, people who are or were connected to the adult-child, and sometimes even a neighbor. Geographical proximity to the family is not required, as support can be conveyed by phone or email. Some supporters who live at a greater distance may attend the session through online video teleconferencing platform such as Zoom, or view a recording of it later on.

When parents object to the idea of rallying support, we recommend that the therapist listen attentively and empathically. A common objection is "the privacy reflex," which is a belief that the parents' and the adult-child's problems are not anyone else's business. Other objections are: the parents' and adult-child's feelings of shame; the fear that disclosure could be traumatic or might risk extreme reactions; and the sense that they have no supporters. The therapeutic challenge is to defuse these objections without alienating the parents.

Sometimes, after the issue of support has been raised, parents tend to skip a session or distance themselves from the intervention. They can be contacted and told that their reservations are important and deserve careful consideration. With highly recalcitrant parents, a middle way can be suggested, in which the supporters are engaged more gradually and as needed. With some families, this gradualist approach led to the recruitment of additional supporters when, for instance, the parents were faced with violence or suicide threats.

A good acquaintance with parents' typical caveats to rallying support can be of great help in increasing the chances of success. We recommend that therapists new to our approach revisit the list of parental reservations provided in Chapter 2. It takes just a few cases to develop a fair proficiency in dealing with such parental objections. We often say to therapists new to the approach that they would win their "NVR badge" after having convened and conducted three supporters' gatherings.

Parents are often reluctant to seek support because they feel that the crushing burden of their total responsibility for their child's well-being cannot be shared with anyone else. Discussing this reluctance, therefore, offers the additional therapeutic value of easing the burden and helping make their inner lives more livable.

In addition to the arguments presented in Chapter 2 in favor of seeking support, practical steps can be taken to help parents obtain it. The therapist asks parents to prepare a list of their relatives and friends, and describe them one by one. This conversation usually leads to a shortlist of potential supporter candidates. The therapist may also offer parents help in writing a letter to these candidates, inviting them to a supporters' session. After receiving this offer, many parents proceed with the invitation on their own. Sometimes, as a result of patient persuasion, a reluctant parental couple would finally agree to invite one supporter. If sensing that the therapeutic alliance is sufficiently robust, the therapist may reply: "Wonderful! Now we need only nine more."

The Supporters' Gathering

The supporters' gathering is often the most important event of the whole treatment. It lifts the veil of secrecy and enhances the family's readiness to consider new options. It relieves parents from the burdens of isolation and strengthens their commitment to action. Supporters' groups in our practice nurture and embrace the entire nuclear family: parents, adult-child and siblings. No parent remains untouched by supporters' expressions of appreciation for their efforts and their child. To maximize these outcomes, however, the therapist must be aware of potential pitfalls.

Supporters are often concerned that the adult-child will feel cornered if approached by a group of people, no matter how well-intentioned. It is recommended that only one or two supporters contact the adult-child in a given week. These contacts should be coordinated with the parents. The therapist briefs supporters on how best to address the adult-child. They are advised to convey to the child their awareness of the problematic events that are taking place at home, and at the same time their affection, readiness to help and belief that the adult-child will overcome the difficulties. A private supporter forum is established via internet platforms such as email or WhatsApp, and both the parents and supporters brief the forum on any problematic or positive events. In this way, the campaign of de-accommodation becomes part of the group's ongoing communication. These briefings can include good news, as well as reports on unpleasant or stressful incidents. The therapist may also participate in the forum, offering their perspective and interpretation of ongoing developments.

Some supporters might feel uncomfortable participating in a group that discusses an adult person's affairs behind the person's back. It should be kept in mind, however, that the supporter gathering is not about the adult-child but about the longstanding crisis in which the parents find themselves. Helping the adult-child is certainly an important motive, but the immediate recipients of support are the parents. The therapist should be aware that some supporters might experience the tension between the parents and adult-child as a conflict of loyalties. For this reason, younger supporters, like the adult-child's friends or siblings, may not be invited to the supporters' gathering. However, this does not mean that they cannot help. With the therapist's guidance, parents learn how to ask for their support. In many cases, help from those younger people proved crucial in conveying to the adult-child that they are not alone. Here is a message from a therapist to the elder sister of a young man, who had voiced reservations about participating in the supporters' meeting (her brother was undergoing an acute manic episode):

I can understand your concern that joining our supporters' meeting might place you in a conflict of loyalties. I would see it as perfectly understandable if you decide not to come. I consider this session as highly urgent because your brother suffers from an acute mental condition, involving high risk. People in such condition may behave in ways that are deeply harmful to themselves and also to others. Those who care for your brother are gathering in order to provide him with a safety net. Many people in your brother's condition react positively to offers of help, sometimes at the very peak of their crisis, sometimes at a later stage. This shows that deep down they know they need help. A lot of research evidence indicates that where a supportive network exists, chances of successfully overcoming the crisis are much higher. Once again, I will respect your decision, if you choose not to participate. Your help can be very meaningful even if you choose not to participate in the meeting itself.

The sister decided not to attend the meeting but asked to be kept in the loop. She became a major positive influence going forward.

Another challenge is when supporters criticize the parents or the adult-child during the meeting. The therapist should politely but assertively counter those comments. Almost always the group will reinforce the therapist's position. In exceptional cases it may be advisable to do without the services of a problematic supporter, for instance a relative who behaves offensively toward the adult-child.

The therapist opens the supporters' gathering by thanking everyone for coming and noting that even a modest contribution can go a long way. Participants are then asked to introduce themselves and say a few words about their relationship with the parents and the adult-child. Most supporters who know the adult-child will compliment their character, thus helping form a positive representation of the adult-child's qualities and capacities. These descriptions often seem surprising to the parents, who sometimes find it hard to see the positive sides of their child because of the difficult home situation. In contrast, it is much easier for people outside the nuclear family to remember the admirable qualities that the adult-child's parents might have forgotten.

This round of self-introductions also allows the therapist to assess which attendees may be best qualified for which supporting role, in terms of their closeness to one family member or another, availability, age and physical distance from the family home. Some participants may be closer to the parents or to one of them and can focus on supporting their wellness. Others may have a special bond with the adult-child, and might be in a position to support the child through what they may experience as a disturbingly radical shift in their life conditions. Others might support the adult-child's siblings, who may have been badly affected by the situation.

After this initial round, the therapist invites the parents to share their difficulties with the group, noting that not all present may be aware of the situation in the family's home. Many parents find this distressing, as they are asked to act against their deep convictions regarding privacy and loyalty and disclose information that they had been hiding, sometimes for years. Faced with this situation, the parents might try to minimize the problem, especially when relating incidents of violence, intimidation and exploitation. The therapist may then respectfully ask the parents to share further details about the harsher moments of their interaction with the adult-child.

At this juncture, details may emerge that had hitherto been kept secret. The forum members, many of whom must have sensed the family's unspoken distress, would finally fathom the depth of its suffering. The problem's "hard core" disclosure often elicits powerful emotional reactions. Participants might cry, become enraged or feel shocked. The therapist's task is to channel these responses to positive ends.

After the parents conclude their disclosure, the therapist summarizes the family's plight, informs the group about the negative impact of accommodation and presents an overview of the therapeutic plan. The parents are then asked to read their announcement draft to the group. The therapist tells the group that the delivery of the announcement marks the beginning of the parents' resistance campaign; that the parents cannot perform their task on their own; and that the supporters can take a critical role in helping the parents successfully cope with their challenge. One simple way to help is by paying visits to the parents and attempting to contact the adult-child. If the adult-child refuses to talk, the supporters are requested to leave a written message. The supporters are told that even a single visit and one email or WhatsApp message to the adult-child can make a difference, especially in the face of violence or other threats. Simply inviting supporters to become involved may have a de-escalating effect.

Our research and experience have shown that the risk of extreme behaviors is substantially reduced when someone from outside the nuclear family is present, either in person or by phone. The therapist concludes this part of the discussion by asking who should contact the adult-child when things at home escalate. At that point, volunteers always come forward.

The focus of supporter gatherings should remain pragmatic and forward-looking. The therapist can stress that continuing accommodation would deeply hurt the adult-child's chances of functioning better. Some supporters may voice concern that their involvement may have adverse effects, for instance the fear that if driven to a corner the adult-child might break down or attempt suicide. The therapist should address these concerns without resorting to blanket reassurances such as "This never happens" or "These suicide threats are only demonstrative." Rather, we would recommend sharing with the group the experience that, when supporters are involved, the risk of extreme acts is reduced. The therapist might also inform the group that they will be available to deal with potential crises.

In the course of the group discussion, often helpful comments arise. Some suggest new possible courses of action. The therapist may propose that some participants would help reduce tensions at home by occasionally inviting the adult-child to stay with them for a while. It is good practice to ask some of the supporters if they would be willing to host the adult-child for a weekend or to help defuse a crisis. In many of our cases, such a respite outside the parental home served as a time-out that led to clear improvements.

Before the gathering is concluded, the therapist invites the supporters to raise any remaining questions or concerns, and proposes that the parents create an email or WhatsApp forum where all present can share information about their contacts with the adult-child.

Guiding the Supporters

In the wake of the supporters' gathering, one or two supporters can contact the adult-child to open a constructive dialogue. Moreover, when there have been violence or threats, a supporter can arrive at the family home. This sets an important precedent; the adult-child now understands that the parents will no longer be alone in extreme situations.

The therapist coordinates the support network. After the email group or WhatsApp forum are set up, the therapist uses it to greet the group and wish it success. Any supporter who has contacted the adult-child is asked to post a short description of the event. During the therapeutic sessions, the therapist and parents occasionally decide together on certain keynote messages. Gradually, a role differentiation emerges.

Some supporters succeed in establishing and maintaining a positive contact with the adult-child. When this proves possible, de-accommodation becomes smoother, less polarized and richer in management options. These supporters can offer mediation, propose joint activities with the adult-child and help create some healthy distancing from the parents. With this type of support, possibilities for study, work or habitation outside the parental home may be explored.

Some group members can serve as buffers against threats and violence. Even if they are not close to the adult-child, their physical presence at the family home in times of escalation conveys that the parents will no longer remain unprotected against the adult-child's outbursts. When the supporters arrive, the adult-child usually retreats to their room. The supporter stays with the parents for a while and leaves a written note for the adult-child. Sometimes, the supporter stays for the night, to ensure the parents' safety. In the wake of such a visit, the chaos usually subsides, sometimes for a long time. The supporter's visit also helps parents to continue de-accommodating.

Phone calls from supporters also help reduce violence. When parents are threatened, they can shut themselves in their room and call for help. In one of our cases, the single mother of a highly impulsive daughter took refuge in a storm shelter with her cell phone. Shortly after, the daughter's phone began ringing. Fifteen minutes later the first supporter arrived. The daughter did not attack her mother again.

Another role for a supporter is that of occupying the house for a few days, to allow the parents to leave for a short break. This role is often taken up by the adult-child's grandparents. A few days away can make parents feel that they can start living again.

The Supportive Role of Other Professionals

An important supportive role is played by professionals, who usually do not participate in the supporters' gathering, but can be contacted at different times. Besides the adult-child's therapist, this role can be also played by the police, a psychiatrist, a social or rehabilitation worker, or a financial consultant.

Most parents are reluctant to involve the police, either because they fear it might cause legal trouble for the adult-child or that it might backfire. We do not recommend or endorse involving the police in communities where such involvement would lead to further escalation or infringement of human rights. However, in cases where there is trust and cooperation between a community and its police force, involving law enforcement officers in conjunction with NVR therapy might be useful. To this end, the therapist may provide the parents with a printed letter, addressed to the police, to be used should they ever feel obliged to call for help, or when neighbors alert the police. The letter explains that the parents came to therapy because of their difficult situation with the adult-child. If the therapist is convinced that the parents are not violent toward the adult-child, this should be stated in the letter. The parents present the letter to the police officer who arrives at the scene. Here is a typical example:

To the police officer,

Alan and Susan, the parents of Mark (17 years old), have consented that I share with you the following: I specialize in counseling to parents who cope with aggressive adolescents. Alan and Susan are consulting with me about their son's school refusal, internet addiction and highly aggressive behavior. I have provided them with this letter in case they would need to ask for police help. In my view, the parents are making every possible effort to cope with the problem in a positive way, so that their son may overcome his difficulties. Based on our consultations, I found the parents to be deeply caring and concerned about Mark, and there is no indication whatsoever of abuse on their part toward him. To my understanding, their request for help should be taken seriously, as their sole wish is that Mark would understand they will do everything possible to protect themselves and help him get better. If it were possible for an officer to reach out for

Mark once again during the upcoming week, chances are that your intervention will have an enduring positive effect.

Sincerely,
[The Therapist]

In our culture, we have found that police involvement in such circumstances
integrates well into our intervention. Sometimes, the police officer sits down
with the adult-child for half an hour or even more. In some of our cases, the
police do as we ask and contact the adult-child several days after the house call.
We have seen very few cases when the mere presence of a police officer did not
calm a violent adult-child, and remove the requirement for actual restraint or
removal to custody. If the adult-child has been diagnosed with a psychiatric
condition, the therapist's letter should mention this. The police will then follow
standard procedure, usually taking the adult-child to a psychiatric emergency
center for evaluation.[2]

Psychiatrists are often involved in the therapeutic program. If an adult-child
was in psychiatric care before the intervention began, the parents' therapist
would inform the psychiatrist and propose an exchange of information. Many
psychiatrists respond willingly to such propositions, as they can greatly benefit
both sides. As for confidentiality, the psychiatrist might ask for the adult-child's
permission to be in contact with the parents' therapist. Adult-children tend to
agree to such requests.

In acute cases, in which the adult-child was not in psychiatric care when the
intervention began, and rejects evaluation or treatment, consultation might still
take place among the psychiatrist, the parents and the therapist, regarding
indications for *compulsory admission*. Sometimes, the adult-child is already a
psychiatric inpatient. In Chapter 6, we describe the special case of a therapeutic
system comprising parents, their therapist and psychiatric caregivers.

Social work and rehabilitation agencies can also support the intervention, by
relieving parents of some of their caregiving burdens and helping them steer
away from the narrative of total responsibility. Workers of such agencies may
offer the adult-child help in joining rehabilitation or assisted living programs.
In a project for parents of adults with HFASD (Golan et al., 2018), elderly
parents of handicapped adult-children were helped to meet with rehabilitation
services and visit their facilities. The parents reported that for the first time they
felt somewhat hopeful about the future.

We occasionally involve financial coaches when an adult-child incurs financial debt and expects the parents to pay it off. In such cases, a major de-
accommodation goal for the parents becomes discontinuing their financial
support, unless the adult-child is willing to undergo financial coaching,

---

[2] Again, this practice is recommended only where there are good police–community relations.

including professional oversight of their financial activities. The coach then develops a financial recovery plan with the adult-child. The parents' financial support is then made conditional on the adult-child's cooperation with the plan. Adult-children who receive such coaching have better chances of becoming financially responsible.

Over and beyond these structured roles and tasks, supporters fulfill important roles that are shaped according to their unique patterns of relating to the adult-child. In the course of our work, we have witnessed an inspiring and infinitely creative variety of support styles that exceeds anything an intervention protocol or a therapist can prescribe. Our more modest role as therapists is just to enable this variety.

The Process of De-Accommodation

Following the announcement and mobilization of supporters, the stage is set for the parents' central mission: reducing accommodation and taking apart the degenerative shelter. This process is vital for allowing a more functional dependence pattern to emerge. The pursuit of functional dependence goes hand in hand with the prevention of escalation. It should be expected that the adult-child will oppose the parents' initiative. This immediate reaction represents an escalation, compared to the relative quiet which the parents might have hitherto been procuring through their accommodation. However, guided by the principles of NVR, parents can substantially reduce this escalation and confine it to the very first stages of the process. As the adult-child understands that the parents are determined not to revert to their former role, and the parents learn to bear the brunt of the adult-child's reaction without giving in or lashing out, escalation subsides.[3]

The following principles guide the process of de-accommodation.

Violent, Destructive and Dangerous Behaviors Come First

Acts and patterns that hurt or endanger the parents, the adult-child or any others should be at the top of the list of resistance and de-accommodation priorities. Typical destructive patterns include suicide threats, physical or emotional violence, vandalism and blackmail. Parents often raise the objection that it would be precisely the project of de-accommodation that would trigger these responses. To them, de-accommodation and extreme risk are two sides of the same coin. One of

---

[3] We've made clear elsewhere (Omer, 2004b; in press) that escalation can be "episodic" or "ongoing." Episodic escalation should be contained in order to prevent immediate harm, such as by bringing in supporters. However, the most damaging kind of escalation is the ongoing kind, which may feed on parental concessions made to avoid episodic escalation. Episodic escalation should not be reduced at the price of the much more damaging ongoing escalation.

our roles as therapists is to help parents separate the two. For example, in dysfunctional bonds a pattern of blackmail often develops, in which threats and services are strictly linked: "If things do not continue as they are, just wait and see what I'll do!" Our goal is to help parents separate these two elements and convey two messages: "We will resist and protect ourselves" and "We will weigh our services in an appropriate way." Appropriate services are those that support improved functioning. Services that impede functioning or harm family life would be phased out. To this end, parents learn that they can protect themselves and reduce their harmful services at the same time. This is precisely the primary goal of NVR.

In order to resist violence in a nonescalating way, it is necessary to lift the veil of secrecy, involve supporters, identify and avoid escalation traps, and accept our inability to control anyone but ourselves. These are key to the intervention. Each act of parental de-accommodation challenges us to revisit these principles and discover how they can apply to the situation. The therapist should discuss each step with parents, planning with them how to implement NVR guidelines regarding secrecy, support, escalation and self-control. Gradually, parents internalize those principles and become capable of implementing them on their own.

Understandably, parents are most fearful when they begin de-accommodating, especially as adult-children react most strongly when their parents begin withholding their services. As parents discover they can rally support, protect themselves and stand their ground, their fear subsides. The more courageous they become, the more the adult-child realizes that the parents are no longer alone, that they can endure the child's extreme moments and that the child can survive their decision to withhold services. But the major discovery that the adult-child makes at the start of this process is that the parents have become able to do the "impossible": to cease accommodating.

Involving Support is Both a Necessary Help and in Itself an Act of De-Accommodation

At first, refusing harmful services may seem to parents like an insurmountable hurdle. To cope with this difficulty, parents are told they can be in touch with the therapist about special problems, or come to extra sessions, if necessary. The supporters play a major role in helping the parents launch this process. For many parents, having a letter for the police at hand may provide an added sense of security. Some parents feel the need to have one or two supporters physically present in their home, as they embark on their de-accommodation program. On very rare occasions, the police are actually involved. All these measures are temporary. The sense of urgency eventually subsides and de-accommodation becomes part of everyday life.

As they start involving supporters, parent often feel as if they were breaching a sacred taboo. The adult-child's explicit or tacit total injunctions regarding secrecy turn the involvement of supporters into a major act of de-accommodation. The introduction of supporters irreversibly changes the family's situation, as a broken secret cannot be unbroken. Moreover, after rallying their support network, parents rarely revert to their previous life in social isolation. In exceptional cases, the adult-child may temporarily move to the house of a relative or friend. Those situations are not only crises but also significant opportunities. Managing them well may speed up the process of de-accommodation.

Victimhood May Be an Act of Accommodation in Itself

Violence is not always a result of the parents' refusal of services but is sometimes part and parcel of "normal" life at the family home. In many cases, parents and their property are routinely subjected to physical violence. Resisting this violence is the foremost task of de-accommodation. Parents are sometimes surprised when we describe their victimhood as a type of harmful service they perform. In effect, parents often serve *themselves* to the adult-child as a punching bag. This service is harmful twice over as it causes enormous suffering to the parents and deeply corrupts the adult-child's character. Few things can corrupt so absolutely as having total power over others. Non-Violent Resistance therefore represents a great hope to parents as well as to adult-children. By resisting violence and oppression, the parents give the adult-child and themselves a real chance.

Apart from Resisting Violence, De-Accommodation Should Be Pursued Gradually

Parents and adult-children alike experience deep anxiety regarding de-accommodation. To cope with this anxiety, and assuming there are no violent or destructive behaviors left to deal with, it is best to proceed gradually, beginning with the lighter tasks and progressing to the heavier ones, as the parents' confidence grows. Three levels of parental de-accommodation can be distinguished, in increasing order of difficulty: (a) reducing services; (b) reducing privacy rights; and, when necessary, (c) changing the adult-child's habitation.

Reducing Services   Although service reduction is considered the easiest of the three task categories, parents may also experience it as difficult. Therefore, we recommend that services are phased out, rather than abruptly discontinued. We also advise that the order and pace of gradual phaseout would be thoroughly discussed with the family, as every family has its own view of the importance and meaning of each service and the costs of discontinuing it.

The following list is not exhaustive, as parental services are infinitely varied.

Laundering, Cooking, Cleaning, Shopping and Transportation. Most parents would agree that providing these services regularly to adult-children can be inappropriate. When these services nurture dysfunctional dependence, reducing or terminating them is a good place to begin. Discussing these services with parents raises important points, such as the parents' narrative of total responsibility, infantilizing beliefs about the adult-child's capabilities, and the parents' tendency to minimize the importance of their own acts. For example, some parents say, "Laundering and cooking are not a problem, I do it for the entire family anyhow" or "Why should I not drive her around? I have time, and if I do not drive her, she will stay in her room." When parents are invited to discuss these beliefs, they may change them. Many parents understand that taking those apparently trivial tasks for granted may harm the adult-child's capacity of functioning.

Financial Services. Reducing financial support for the adult-child is a major act of de-accommodation. Many parents pay their adult-child a monthly allowance, often by direct bank transfer. The allowance can be reduced toward complete termination within a few months. Other financial services include paying for the adult-child's clothing, entertainment, travel, addictions, traffic fines, automobile expenses, personal or business debts, or lawyers' fees.

Supporters can help parents overcome the stress that is linked to financial de-accommodation by offering advice to the adult-child on how to develop a financial recovery plan, or by developing a group policy of no loans, should the adult-child ask group members for financial help. In case the parents had covered any outstanding bank loans the adult-child had in the past, both the bank and the child should be notified that this will not happen again. Parents sometime intervene to rescue their child from losing their credit card. We tell the parents that losing the credit card is an important consequence that the adult-child should endure on the way toward financial responsibility.

Internet and Cellular Connectivity. Many parents and adult-children consider internet and cellular access as the most self-evident service. Discontinuing the child's internet or cellular package payments, or transferring the cell phone's account to the adult-child's name can be small but highly symbolic steps. In case the adult-child is addicted to the Internet, the parents may have to take more radical measures.[4]

---

[4] See Chapter 5.

Complying with Problematic Habits. Many parents cooperate with their adult-children's dysfunctional habits, participating in compulsive rituals or allowing them to take their meals in their rooms. To resist this, parents often find it necessary to reduce privacy rights (see below).

Allowing the Adult-Child to Abuse or Take Control of the Family Home and Facilities. There are different ways in which adult-children use the family home for their own problematic ends and to detriment of other family members. A typical situation is that of adult-children who leave their room only at night for a noisily prepared nocturnal meal, leaving a mess in the kitchen. Some adult-children colonize family areas, occasionally even declaring them "off limits" to siblings or parents. Adult-children who have OCD sometimes use the family home as a staging area for compulsive rituals or as a hoarding depot. Others host parties when the parents are away and consume their alcohol. Support is of course critical in the parents' attempt to take back their home.

Serving the Adult-Child's Need for Unlimited Reassurance or Accommodating to Blaming Outbursts. Many parents make themselves available around the clock to provide unlimited reassurance to the adult-child. Continuous reassurance is one form of accommodation implicated in the perpetuation of anxiety disorders (Shimshoni et al., 2019). Parents can be helped to cease continuously reassuring their children. Some adopt a standard phrase such as, "You know what I think. I will not discuss this with you again" or, "I'll give you a short answer once. After that I will not answer." Some resort to the step of announcing to the adult-child that they would limit themselves to one short conversation per day, declining further phone calls from the adult-child for 24 hours.

A particularly offensive interaction is the staging of ritualistic blaming binges, in which parents are repeatedly accused of having shaped the adult-child into what they are today, with the implication that the parents have to pay the price. Regardless of what parents did or did not do in the past that harmed their children, they are helped to understand that an unbounded receptiveness to these accusations is in itself deeply harmful both to themselves and to the adult-child. They become willing to protect themselves, limit their response to these ruminations and involve supporters in resisting them. Parents announce they will no longer take part in these conversations and will immediately forward any blaming text messages to a supporter who has been designated to respond on their behalf. Instead of getting an answer from their parents, the adult-child receives an answer from a supporter. Thereupon, this kind of negative communication dwindles.

Each of these steps to parental de-accommodation may raise the parents' anxiety. The therapist's role is to address the parents' concerns, and help them prepare for what might happen. This discussion often revisits issues that had been considered earlier in the therapy; however, this time it refers to more specific acts of de-accommodation. The pragmatic focus of the current intervention stage allows parents to overcome their anxiety better than the earlier, more general, discussions. When those discussions take place while de-accommodation is underway, the parents' sense of foreboding is gradually transformed into a sense of coping.

Adult-children react differently to their parents' decision to reduce services. Some try to suppress the parents' "rebellion" by rage, vandalizing the home or threatening suicide. Some accuse parents of having betrayed them and claim that the parents' new approach will only make everything worse. Others try to delay, saying they do want to become independent but that this would take time, they want to do it at their own pace and the parents' de-accommodation acts are only making it worse. Some react by pretending to ignore the parents' steps, withdrawing into their room or remaining in bed. Whatever the response, and given that parents are sufficiently determined and consistent, adult-children realize that the wheels have been set in motion and that the refuge they had constructed for themselves will not be the same. The parents' refusal to accommodate gains momentum, especially as the parents become ready to stop seeing the adult-child's room as sacrosanct.

Reducing Privacy Rights   Breaking taboos requires courage, but after breaking the first, it is easier to break the next. The parents have already crossed the sacrosanct line of absolute privacy in involving supporters. This breach is made evident in the adult-child's protest, "How dare you talk to strangers about my private life?" To help the parents withstand the adult-child's anger, the therapist discusses with them the fact that privacy is not an absolute value but one among other values. Privacy should be respected but only so long as it is not used in destructive ways. Society reserves to itself the right to waive privacy rights in cases of violent behaviors, for instance domestic violence. The same rule is valid when the child abuses the parents or siblings or uses their own private space for self-destructive activities.

Breaking the secrecy taboo by involving supporters usually arouses considerable anger. The immediate result may be that the adult-child boycotts the parents and some of the supporters. Usually, however, the adult-child stays in contact with one or two selected supporters. Little by little, the boycott is rescinded, especially as the parents and the supporters respond to the adult-child in positive ways.

The next level of reduction in privacy rights regards the adult-child's room, which is usually a mess. Many of those rooms are filled up with piles of clothes, papers, empty food containers and filth. Many adult-children not only refuse to clean their room but also forbid anybody else to do so. Any attempt by the parents to change this situation meets with furious resistance. If they somehow manage to step in, they are met by the outraged command, "Get out of *my* room!"

Parents are often stunned into silence by this affirmation of an absolute right. Many say, "But she is right. This is her room." The therapist should then answer, "It is not just her room. It is her room in *your* house." In other words, the child's room is theirs not in the sense of unalienable property but in a conditional sense, as a right that is conceded by the parents upon fulfillment of certain conditions. Almost all parents agree that their child's right to the room should be respected only so long as the room is not used destructively. If this condition is violated, the parents not only have the right but also the duty to rescind the adult-child's absolute right to privacy in their room. This understanding allows for the formulation of a plan on how to reduce the adult-child's pernicious privacy.

Our first recommendation is that the parents enter the adult-child's room three times a day, for about 10 minutes at a time. They can try to engage in conversation or remain silent. If the adult-child asks the parents what they are doing, the parents can say, "Your room is part of our house." It is not necessary to explain further. They should stay in the room for the planned 10 minutes, even if the adult-child leaves the room. They can use the time to bring some order to the chaos or write a message that they leave on the computer desk. These actions are reminders of parental presence. The adult-child often protests that it is their house too. The parents may then say, "You are our child and you are welcome to live with us. But this is our house." To some parents, this message does not come easily.

This reluctance may serve as a cue for the therapist to discuss how the parents have become effaced and how important it is for them to reassert their presence, voice and rights. In the end, virtually all parents succeed not only in saying that the house is theirs but also in identifying themselves with that simple truth.

If the door to the room is locked and the adult-child refuses to allow the parents to enter, it may be necessary to remove the lock. This requires the help of supporters. The supporters can tell the adult-child that if they keep the door locked, the parents will remove it. Thereupon, some adult-children agree reluctantly to keep the door unlocked. If the adult-child barricades themselves by placing furniture against the door, the parents remove the door. This may serve as a temporary arrangement or may lead to the adult-child's deciding to move out. The supporters can help in this transition, for instance by offering the adult-child a temporary place to stay. Invariably, the adult-child behaves in a much more mature way in the supporters' house. The transitional lodgings are thus an important step toward more functional dependence. The stay at a relative's house is usually limited, serving as a transition phase to a more permanent solution. During this period, the adult-child's hosts should be invited to participate in one or more treatment sessions. In all the cases we have treated, a temporary move to another house has proven quite beneficial.

Parents are often amazed by how the adult-child can be cordial, considerate and pleasant with others while behaving horribly toward them. In the rare cases in which the adult-child also behaves unacceptably in the relatives' home, other supporters can be involved; this usually leads to rapid improvement. It is as if the adult-child's dysfunctional ways of behaving did not have time to take root in the new surroundings, remaining much more responsive to external influences than in the parental home.

In most cases, however, the parents' visits to the adult-child's room do not result in a change of lodging. The adult-child sometimes reacts by leaving the room and trying to ignore the parents' presence. Sometimes, the adult-child may vandalize the parents' room. The parents are then helped to deploy a tenacious effort of Non-Violent Resistance. They document the wreckage and involve supporters, the social services or the police. This stance puts a stop to the violence and makes way for a negotiation of new rules.

Changing the Habitation As the parents reduce services and, if necessary, privacy rights, many adult-children improve their functioning. Violence, humiliation and escalation diminish. The positive sides of the relationship, which had previously been in abeyance, reappear. Many adult-children begin to participate in household chores and costs. Others start studying, working and socializing. Sometimes, however, functioning does not improve. The adult-child seems to take the parents' moves in their stride, remaining entrenched in deep passivity. It may then be necessary to move to the next level and get the adult-child to leave the house.

Helping the parents to this major decision takes patience, tact and empathy. Most parents know that the adult-child can function better outside the parental home. In many cases, the adult-child had done so in the past. In some cases, the return to the parental home was indicative of a steep drop in the adult-child's functioning. For the more resilient, a temporary return to the parents' home in the wake of life changes (e.g., graduation, the end of a marriage, loss of a job or discharge from the military) may serve as a recovery period. However, for the adult-children we are concerned with, the parental home may not at all be a stepping-stone. As in nature, some chicks leave the nest on their own but some must be helped out. For some parents, the act of launching may seem like an expulsion. Initially, at least, they react with horror at the very mention of that possibility: "What, should I throw her out of the house?"

Ending the adult-child's stay in the parental home is of course the heavier option in the process of de-accommodation. This step will not be undertaken unless the options of reducing services and privacy rights have been exhausted. In weighing the need for separate lodgings, the therapist and the parents should ask themselves several questions: Did the former steps lead to a more functional dependence? Are there signs of progress in the adult-child's relationship with other family members, participation in house maintenance, socializing or looking for work? Under those conditions, there is no reason to push. The processes may lead either to the adult-child leaving the house on their own initiative or to normalizing the situation to a degree in which cohabitation becomes an acceptable way of life. However, absence of progress or continuing self-entrenchment suggest that the heart of the problem lies in the cohabitation of the parents and the adult-child. In this case, the accommodation element that remains to be dismantled is the cohabitation itself.

The parents should formally notify the adult-child that they no longer want them living in their home. It is recommended that they be sincere, saying: "We believe that so long as you live with us, you will remain totally dependent on us. We do not know if you will function better outside the home. However, we do not want to be the ones that provide you with the conditions to remain passive." This is very different from "We are doing this for your own good!" Such a declaration would probably provoke further opposition, as nobody wants to be told by others what is, or is not, for their own good. The more limited message, that the parents do not want to be those that enable the adult-child's continued passivity, is harder to reject. Even if the adult-child implies that they do not care, the parents may feel and show that they do. As last resort, the parents may share another truth with their adult-child: "Even if you don't agree with us, we no longer want to share our living quarters with anyone on a permanent basis. We are 60+, our needs and preferences have changed, and we need our own quiet and privacy."

The parents then tell the adult-child either directly or through a mediator that they will not withhold their parental help and support. However, that help will take new forms. The therapist discusses the ways in which the parents may help the adult-child find and possibly pay for a new place to live. This discussion is very important in addressing the parents' feeling that they are throwing their child out. Their readiness to help, directly or through supporters, turns the "throwing out" into an "easing out." The parents do not need the adult-child's consent. They take steps to end the cohabitation.

Many parents wonder what they can do if the adult-child simply refuses to move out. Based on numerous cases, we can answer that this rarely happens. When parents are truly ripe for sending off their adult-children, adult-children rarely stick around. In the unlikely event that refusal persists, supporters can be brought in to tell the adult-child that they are willing to help but that the child must leave. In some very rare cases, social services or the police should be involved. Almost invariably, the adult-child ends up leaving the parental home. In some of our cases, the parents moved into another house that had no space for the adult-child.

Sometimes, the adult-child started to behave more functionally in reaction to the parents' steps to get them out of the house. In some cases, a point of equilibrium was reached in which dysfunctional dependence was reduced to the extent that the parents were willing to reconsider their decision. However, with the help of supporters they made it clear to the adult-child that they would not go back to the previous situation.

The decision to end the cohabitation sometimes leads to additional changes. Some adult-children finally agree to get psychiatric help, which to that point they had adamantly refused. Some convince their parents that things are improving by finding work. More frequently, however, the decision to get the adult-child to leave the parental home became a reality within a few months to one year.

Therapy continues after the adult-child leaves the parental home. It is important to assuage the parents' anxiety about the adult-child and the kind of assistance they should or should not provide. Some parents constantly buy food for the adult-child, even to the point of stocking the refrigerator. Some parents become extremely worried about how the adult-child spends their free time and try to get information from neighbors or friends. Dealing with those reactions and further reducing accommodation can be an important therapeutic task. Some adult-children, especially the more functional ones, keep their activities hidden from the parents. They sometimes say that the parents should mind their own business. This legitimate desire for privacy after leaving the parental home may also be due to resentment or anger. By keeping the parents in the dark, they may be punishing them for pushing them out. In many cases, this anger eventually subsides, making room for a closer relationship. In one of our cases the 28-year-old son invited the parents for a "house warming," four years after he was living in his own apartment!

The Conclusion Stage

Non-Violent Resistance therapy for AED has an open-ended conclusion. Monthly or bimonthly follow-up sessions are recommended for a while. The therapist should discuss with the parents under what circumstances they should come for a short-term renewal of therapy. For example, if the adult-child has a crisis, is hospitalized, stops working or makes extraordinary requests for money, this may create high pressure to reestablish dysfunctional dependence. Those eventualities should be discussed during the conclusion stage.

Usually, therapy approaches its end when a point of equilibrium is reached, in which dysfunctional dependence gives way to more functional patterns. This could mean that the violence and emotional blackmail stops, accommodation services are reduced and the adult-child resumes some normative occupational and social activities. Alternatively, therapy ends when the adult-child leaves the parental home, the parents cope with the ensuing anxiety and resist falling back into the trap of accommodation. An important consideration when the adult-child continues living in the parental home is whether the home is no longer a degenerative shelter. This means that the adult-child takes some part in the family's activities, is no longer locked in their room and the room is no longer a place to hide but part of the house. It is important to review these changes with the parents. Parents should be trained to recognize signs of danger, so that they can react to them in time. Optimally, the parents and the therapist make a joint decision to stop the therapy. Sometimes, after some progress has been made, the parents cancel a meeting and fail to reschedule. In such circumstances, the therapist should request one more session to discuss what has been achieved and how to prevent untoward developments. We do not believe that the therapist's role is to try to convince the parents to remain in therapy. Even if the therapist thinks that the conclusion is premature, it is better to view the parents' wish to stop as expressing their need for a well-earned respite.

A good way to review the parents' accomplishments is to read with them the notes of the first therapy session. This helps give the parents a good perspective on their capacity to resist and de-accommodate, as well as on the adult-child's capacity to function. Reflecting on what had brought the parents into the first meeting also gives them a clear reminder about what should be prevented.

However, not all treatments come to a happy ending. Some parents come to one or two sessions and conclude that this kind of therapy is not for them or that they are still not ready. Sometimes, even though the parents seem willing, the therapy plods on without real action. This is often because one or both parents is unwilling to de-accommodate. If the therapist's attempts at persuasion fail, it may be advisable to tell the parents that, for the time being at least, progress does not seem possible. Sometimes, this candid admission shocks the parents into taking some initial steps that put the therapy back on course. All in all, the proportion of parents that fail to be engaged or give up in the middle is low.

We would like to conclude by reviewing what positive changes can be expected, if the practical steps described in this chapter are undertaken:

> As parents provide fewer age-inappropriate services, the adult-child becomes more functional.
>
> As parents become better able to resist, the child's use of violence, blackmail and humiliation decreases.
>
> As parents improve their self-control, there are fewer clashes.
>
> As parents stop justifying themselves or undertaking steps to appease their sense of guilt, there is less blaming.
>
> As parents focus more on their own needs, the adult-child acts more in ways that acknowledge those needs.

As parents engage less in continuous reassurance, the adult-child develops better ways to regulate their own emotions.

As parents relinquish their wish to direct the adult-child's life, the adult-child develops better ways to direct their own life.

As parents learn to cope with shame and lift the veil of secrecy, they and the adult-child become less isolated.

As parents become able to get support, their helplessness and impulsiveness is reduced.

As parents stop telling the adult-child what to think, feel or do, the adult-child becomes more able to think, feel and act by themselves.

4   Suicide Threats

Our son is 26. He does not work or study. He lives at home and spends almost all of his time cloistered in his room. He avoids conversing with us, and responds only with monosyllables when we address him. If we ask him about his plans for the future, he tells us to leave him alone, that he is not even sure he wants to go on living and that by pressuring him we only bring him closer to the edge.

Our 16-year old daughter has tried to commit suicide. Although she has friends and is a good student, lately she has become withdrawn, cries a lot and paints deeply frightening pictures. She posted a message in Facebook, saying goodbye to her friends. A friend of hers felt concerned and called us. We looked for her and found her in the basement, tying a nylon rope to a hook on the ceiling.

Our 24-year old daughter studied to be a teacher and has worked for two years in a primary school. She left her job a year ago and is not looking for a new one. She lives at home but does not help with the housework or participate in the life of the family. She says she cannot find herself in the extremely competitive world outside. Every time we think about demanding she find a job, we start worrying that she might hurt herself.

These cases illustrate the different forms in which suicide threats appear in the families we are treating. The first is a general threat used to keep parents at bay. The second is a serious attempt, which the parents managed to stop in the last moment. The third involves no explicit threat, but the parents are concerned in ways that make them reduce their demands.

There are various dimensions that may be considered in such cases. The first is the dimension of suicide risk. There is a vast literature on suicidality, particularly among the young, aiming at defining valid indicators of suicide risk and strategies for reducing it (e.g., Adrian, 2018; Gold & Frierson, 2020). The second is the dimension linking suicide risk to the quality of the parent–child relationship, and proposing therapeutic interventions to improve the relationship, thus reducing the risk. Major contributions of this kind were made from the perspective of Dialectical Behavior Therapy (Miller et al., 2017) and from Attachment Based Family Therapy (Diamond et al., 2010; 2012). The third is the dimension of how the perception of suicide threat by the parents may lead them to increase their accommodation, and how many adult-children may influence the parents' sense of threat by explicit or implicit communications. This third dimension is what we term the *context of intimidation*. We found few studies or interventions designed to deal with this dimension (Omer & Dolberger, 2015). That is the purpose of the present chapter.

Our approach aims at helping parents reduce both the power and the risk posed by suicide threats in the third sense described above. By "power," we mean the coercive influence exerted by the threat in cowing the parents into submission and poisoning the family atmosphere. Many parents believe that complying with the adult-child's expectations is the only way to reduce suicide risk. In their minds, there is no way to counter both the coercion and the risk. Our position is the opposite: The best way to reduce suicide risk is also the best way to reduce the coercion.

One important link between the coercive power of suicide threats and suicide risk is that parental compliance leads to escalation. Bateson's (1972) classical analysis led to the understanding that escalation can be *symmetrical* or *complementary*. In symmetrical escalation, the two sides reflect each other: Shouts lead to shouts, blows to blows and threats to threats. The conflict escalates, as each side believes it has to shout, threaten or hit more than the other. Complementary escalation follows the logic of blackmail: Complying with the threat increases the risk that the blackmailer will raise both the demands and the threats that are needed to guarantee the victim's continued compliance. The danger of this dual escalation is greater than the sum of its parts, for symmetrical and complementary escalation fuel each other. Thus, the continuous frustration of submission leads to outbursts against the blackmailing party, triggering bouts of symmetrical escalation. As a result, the stakes keep rising. The only way to stop the spiral is to resist the threat in a nonescalating way. That is precisely the goal of NVR.

Another reason why giving in to suicide threats tends to augment the risk of suicide is that accommodation deepens dysfunction. As the adult-child becomes less able to function, despair and isolation deepen. Accommodation feeds helplessness and loneliness, gradually driving the adult-child toward the brink. Our goal is to reverse this malignant process.

The very nature of a suicidal crisis may justify the involvement of supporters in a family system that was previously impermeable to outside help. Although the adult-child may react angrily, the availability of support changes the family constellation. Parents may initially be concerned about the child's reaction but this changes rapidly, as supporters help contain destructive reactions. We know of no single case in which the planned involvement of supporters provoked a suicide attempt. In contrast, risk increases so long as the family remains sealed in its bubble.

There is another reason why the shadow of suicide hovers continuously over families with a pattern of dysfunctional dependence. The dependence bond consists of countless "rescue acts." The core of the bond is a deep belief linking the child's subsistence to the acts the parents feel obliged to perform. The parents see themselves as sustaining their child's very existence. Commonplace questions in other families such as "Shall we go to the movies?" or "Where shall we plan our holiday?" may be experienced as questions of life and death. Helping the parents free themselves from this intolerable burden is a major goal in our work. One of the rewards of completing the NVR program is the parents' relief when they become able to do small things that in other families are taken for granted.

The NVR Program for Suicide Threats

The NVR program is relevant for (a) explicit threats that emerge in a context of intimidation (e.g., an adolescent threatens that unless the parents act in a given way she will kill herself), (b) implicit threats (e.g., an adult-child hints that if his seclusion is disturbed, life may become an impossible burden) or (c) the parents are afraid that any change in their accommodation practices may bring their child to the brink, even if the child never alluded to this possibility. In this situation, we may talk of "intimidation" without an "intimidator." The parents play both roles in the process: They raise the specter of suicide and react to it, without any active involvement by the child.

The presence of intimidation, even of the most explicit form, does not necessarily mean that the threat is merely demonstrative. We believe that any threat represents a risk and that dismissing it may intensify the risk. In NVR, parents are helped to respond to threats in ways that do not label them as demonstrative and yet counter their coercive power.

A suicide threat is uniquely compelling, for it threatens to stop not only the present interaction but all future ones. It is literally the "last word." We view suicide threats as the most violent form of communication. The fact that the intended object of violence is the child who issues the threat does not, in any way, diminish the violence of the message. At one stroke, the child threatens to destroy their own life and that of their parents.

Parents often react to suicide threats by panicking, lashing out, dismissing the threat or remaining passive. These reactions have several drawbacks. Panicking increases arousal and dyscontrol (Lebowitz & Omer, 2013); lashing out or giving in escalates the conflict (Omer, 2004b; in press); and remaining passive, ignoring or minimizing the threat leaves the child feeling unsupported. All these parental reactions have been linked to suicide risk (Daniel & Goldston, 2009; Dube et al., 2001; Fergusson et al., 2000; Johnson et al., 2002; Wagner et al., 2003).

Most programs that involve parents are geared to improving family communication, increasing positive interactions and strengthening the parent–child bond (e.g., Diamond et al., 2010; 2012; Hooven, 2013; Stanley et al., 2009).

These goals are important, as the literature has shown that suicidal children and their parents have serious deficits in those areas (Kashani et al., 1989; Wagner et al., 2003). However, we think that these programs fail to address a number of problems that are highly frequent in AED. Thus, adult-children who threaten suicide often refuse to come to treatment (Carlton & Deane, 2000; Wyman et al., 2008); parents are in deep distress and should be considered as clients in their own right; and little attention is given to the threat-interaction as a risk factor in itself and to the question of how parents can reduce its destructive potential (an important exception is Dialectical Behavior Therapy, e.g., Ben-Porath, 2010; Miller et al., 2017).

In the mind of a person who is threatening suicide, there is an internal debate over life versus death. Shneidman's (1985) seminal theory of suicide is based on this premise. He situates this inner dialogue in "the parliament of the mind." He assumed that so long as suicide is not completed, the voices arguing for life are still probably dominant. Attacking the person, remaining passive or ignoring the threat might strengthen the "suicidal faction" in the parliament of the mind.

The urgency of suicide threats requires a two-phase approach: a *containment phase* in which parents cope with the immediate crisis, followed by an *anchoring phase* in which parents anchor themselves in their parental role and support system in ways that increase their child's stability. NVR fosters containment and anchoring by promoting the following processes.

From Helplessness to Presence

Parents often feel paralyzed, have an emotional outburst, submit to the threat or try to ignore it. The helplessness reflected in those reactions may have very negative effects: the child feels abandoned, the conflict escalates and dysfunctional patterns are perpetuated. However, if parents act in ways that convey presence instead of helplessness, the crisis can be contained and the basis laid for further improvement.

The containment phase is launched by an announcement in which the parents communicate to the child their decision to remain present in the child's life and resist suicide to the best of their abilities. This announcement is delivered in a similar manner to the announcement that we described in Chapter 3. It is helpful to have a supporter nearby when delivering it. Here is an illustrative text:

Dear Emmy,

We decided to do all in our power to resist suicide and support you in your trouble. We know you are suffering and will do our best to stand by you. We will not remain distant or uninvolved but be as close as we can. We will no longer keep this secret but get help from anybody who is willing to help us. We feel that getting help is our utmost duty, for life and death are not private issues. We know that we will go through a difficult period but we will be together in this.

Your loving parents

The shift from helplessness to presence is manifested by an increase in contact. If the threat is especially urgent (e.g., if there are signs of actual preparations or an attempt was already made), parents are requested to set up a suicide watch, not only to prevent the attempt, but also as a manifestation of caring presence. The suicide watch sends a message that "We are here and will stay here to the best of our abilities." Parents often object that they cannot keep the watch forever and that, once the child is left alone, the risk of suicide will rise again. Indeed, it is impossible to be on permanent suicide watch. However, the suicide watch conveys a message of care and involvement that reduces the child's sense of isolation. This experience is intensified when the people on watch are relatives and friends, who take shifts. An adolescent or young adult who experiences the devotion of a group of people who are willing to stand by their side for hours and days will feel less abandoned. The sense of connectedness that is engendered by this experience can overcome the wish to die.

The gradual transition from containment to anchoring can be illustrated by the passage from an intense suicide watch into a more virtual manifestation of presence (e.g., by means of constant telephone contacts or text messages). When parents succeed in becoming present to a child's mind in situations of risk, the risk diminishes (Omer, 2017). By their very presence, the parents and supporters strengthen the child against the temptation of suicide. The intense presence of the first phase conveys the message of containment. The presence that is achieved by multiple caring messages from different sources conveys anchoring. The transition from containment to anchoring may be likened to a progressive lengthening of the anchor rope: the child remains connected to the anchor, but in a manner that leaves more room for movement.

From Isolation to Support

Keeping the threat secret drastically reduces connectedness. Secrecy is detrimental for both child and parents because the parents remain maximally vulnerable to emotional blackmail, possibilities of assistance are restricted and the recursive aspects of the suicide interaction are perpetuated. Secrecy and isolation nurture suicide threats. In contrast, lifting the veil of secrecy and involving a network of supporters often leads to a swift change in the conditions that maintain suicidal dynamics.

The positive influence of support on suicide risk has been demonstrated by research. In one remarkable study (King et al., 2019), adolescents who were hospitalized for attempted suicide were asked to nominate "caring adults" who they thought would be supportive after they are discharged. These supportive persons were encouraged to maintain weekly contact with the youths. Dramatic mortality differences were found between this group and controls that did not receive this treatment, 11 to 14 years after index hospitalization. Such a procedure might also be possible in some of our cases; however, many adult-children would not comply with such a request. The parents would then be the ones who choose the supporters. In our experience many adult-children are willing to accept help from supporters they did not choose.

Many parents who had formerly been reluctant to contact supporters change their minds when faced with a suicide threat, because in those situations the right to privacy is relegated to the back seat. The supporters have no difficulty making this clear, for instance by saying to the adult-child: "Of course we were notified! It is a question of life and death!" or "If your parents kept this secret, it is as if they were giving up on you! Neither they nor we are ready to give up on you!"

The voicing of a suicide threat can be a turning point in therapy. To turn the crisis into an opportunity, parents must be helped, so that they can clearly communicate their need for support to their potential helpers. The following message, transmitted both verbally and as text message, was sent by the parents of an adolescent to some potential supporters:

Dear [Supporter's Name],

Our daughter Mary threatened to commit suicide, if we insist that she returns to school. This is the first time we have decided to ask for help. We are now in parent-therapy, where we are learning to overcome helplessness and isolation. We understand that by remaining alone and maintaining secrecy, we were making things worse. So, we decided to invite you to a supporters' meeting. In the meantime, we are setting up a suicide watch, so as not to leave Mary alone. We are also developing a plan how not to give in to Mary's threat, but help her return to school as soon as possible. We would be very grateful if you could visit us during this week and, if Mary agrees, have a conversation with her. If she doesn't agree, you could leave her a short message. In any case, your visit will be enormously important for us.

Yours, Silvia and Jack

The creation of a supporters' network is crucial not only for the containment phase, but also for facilitating the transition to the anchoring phase. The involvement of supporters in the suicidal crisis makes it more likely for parents to seek help with other, less urgent, problems, which are more typical of the anchoring phase. The availability of a support system enables parents to anchor themselves in their parental role. In this respect, the anchor metaphor is especially apt: A small anchor can stabilize a relatively large ship on account of its spikes (the supporters); an anchor with only one spike (the isolated parent) would be much less effective.

From Submission to Resistance

In families with an adult-child, the suicide threat is almost always the last link in a chain of interactions based on coercive and dysfunctional demands. The suicide threat is the logical conclusion. The message, "If you don't do this for me, I cannot live!" epitomizes the dysfunctional dependence bond.

It may sound counterintuitive that, precisely when an adult-child threatens suicide, parents should resist demands they had ordinarily complied with. However, our experience has shown that a suicide threat can open a unique window for change. Its very extremity legitimizes breaking the patterns that led to it. The threat demonstrates to the parents how destructive accommodation can be. Any attempt to counter the threat without changing the coercion–accommodation pattern makes the next threat more likely.

Parents become able to resist if they are supported, and support becomes readily available because of the suicide threat. Some supporters are requested to contact the child soon after the announcement. Sometimes, one or more supporters are already in the house. Parents may tell the child, "We have already notified some people who are close to us. Uncle Steve is now in the dining room and is aware of what is going on." Supporters thus become witnesses and validators of the rite of transition signaled by the announcement. When there has already been an attempted suicide, supporters can come to the hospital[1] or visit the child at home, thus conveying that the situation has changed.

Resistance is also manifested against the suicide intention itself. To be effective, resistance should not take the form of a moral admonishment but that of an existentially engaging encounter. The therapist asks the parents about the people who matter most to the child. Those people are then asked to visit the child, openly discuss the suicide intention with them and even "beg for the child's life."

Typical candidates for this role are grandparents, uncles, siblings and friends. We do not rule out including young children among the suppliants, especially if

---

[1] Hospital visits are a special occasion. The adult-child can hardly refuse them, as the supporters are showing their care and concern in a socially sanctioned manner. The hospital visit also serves as the prologue to later home visits. In this way, hospital visits can be the perfect gateway for involving supporters without arousing resistance.

an actual suicide attempt has been made. We reject the objection that this would be psychologically cruel for the young child; the suicide of a loved one would be even more so. In addition, siblings are often witnesses to suicide threats. Therefore, involving them in the intervention helps them no less than it does the parents. We believe that including siblings by providing them with clear and age-appropriate information gives them a constructive role in the suicidal crisis. This is far better than keeping them in the role of presumably uninformed bystanders.

Sixteen-year-old Ann (mentioned at the beginning of this chapter) was sent to a psychiatric ward after her suicide attempt. When she was discharged after a few weeks, her parents were in deep anxiety and came to us for treatment. Their therapist asked them which people were the most significant in Ann's life. The parents immediately mentioned her grandmother and her 12-year-old brother, Arthur. They were both invited to a session with the parents. Neither had been informed about what had happened to Ann, although Arthur had asked the parents and gotten no answer. The therapist helped the parents to come clean with them. He then explained that Ann might be helped by a direct appeal from them, since they were closest to her. The therapist coached them to speak openly to Ann and, if necessary, to beg for her life. He also told them not to scold her, but to speak in a loving and caring tone. Arthur asked to be left alone with Ann. After about 15 minutes, the parents knocked on the door to find sister and brother crying in each other's arms. Ann swore she would never try to kill herself again.

The parental experience of being able to withstand the child's dysfunctional demands in a suicidal crisis can be invaluable in helping them discontinue a longstanding pattern of accommodation and submission. However, those gains are not automatic. Many parents revert to their familiar routine once the crisis is over. To prevent this, care must be taken to transform containment into anchoring. Parents must be helped to recognize the connection between their accommodating behaviors and the suicidal crisis. The message to the parents is, "If you could avoid submitting under the threat of suicide, you definitely can do it under less extreme conditions." The suicide crisis may thus become an opportunity to end a host of inappropriate services. Learning they can withstand the pressure of a suicide threat becomes a self-anchoring experience that helps the parents to stabilize themselves in other situations (Omer et al., 2013).

From Escalation to Self-Control

Suicide threats do not come from out of the blue; they are preceded by an emotional crescendo unwittingly fanned by parental reactions. Those parents often get caught in a double pattern of symmetrical and complementary escalation. Non-Violent Resistance helps them to recognize and avoid this pattern. During sessions, situations of escalation are examined and reactions that manifest self-control are proposed and rehearsed.

Emphasizing self-control rather than control over others may foster a positive change in the suicidal tug-of-war. Parents are encouraged to tell the adult-child, "We will do all in our power to prevent you from killing yourself. But we know we cannot control you." The compulsion to control is thus replaced by the duty to resist. In resisting, we do not have control over the other. But the positive strength conveyed by the acts of resistance more than outweighs the parents' admission that they have no control over what the adult-child does.

The message of persistence ("You don't have to win but only to persist.") adds the factor of time to the renunciation of control. This message is a good antidote to the sense of absolute urgency that fuels the suicidal dynamics. The parents react to messages like, "Do this or I'll kill myself!" by saying, "We will stand by you today, tomorrow and the day after." They learn to take a deep breath and to think not in terms of hours or days but weeks and months. Actually, NVR is effective with both time frames. Parents are helped to act decidedly in the here and now but in ways that convey long-term endurance and self-control, rather than panic, anger or helplessness.

In the interactions that characterize the dependence bond, the adult-child's sense of urgency is multiplied by that of the parents. Instead of an alliance between the child and the parents, there is an "alliance of urgencies," a mutual spiral of suicidal panic. In NVR, in contrast, the suicidal urge is no longer viewed as a fire that must be put out immediately but as a fever that must be endured until it breaks. However, the parents should not tell the child, "You can endure the pain." but rather, "We will stay with you and get through this together." They thus share some of their own power of endurance with their child.

From Distancing and Hostility to Care and Support

Non-Violent Resistance does not limit itself to struggling against violent, oppressive and destructive acts but involves expressions of respect and care. This is true even in the sociopolitical sphere and infinitely more so in the application of NVR to the family. Helping parents to express care and respect can have a life-enhancing influence on the "parliament of the mind" (Shneidman, 1985). Sometimes, however, parents feel inhibited in their ability to do so because the process of mutual distancing and hostility may *block the caring dialogue* (Jakob, 2019). A common reason for parents' inability to express positive feelings is their expectation that the child will ignore or blatantly reject them.

In our program, parents are helped to take steps that express care, respect and reconciliation, even while expecting a possible negative reaction. They are encouraged to deliver one-sided positive messages in writing, give the child symbolic gifts or propose a joint activity that they used to enjoy. The parents are explicitly prepared for the child's possible rejection. They may then say, "I am doing this because I care for you, but I cannot force you to accept it."

A mother baked a cake for her 16-year-old son who was so addicted to a computer game that he had threatened to kill himself if she interrupted him again while he was playing. She knocked on his door and said, "I made you a coconut cake." As he cursed at her and her cake through the closed door, she answered, "I made it for you because I love you, but I can't force you to eat it. It will be in the fridge, just for you." She thus put her son in the dilemma of being tough and passing up the cake, or swallowing his pride and eating it. The dilemma was made even harder, as the mother baked another cake after a week and again after two weeks. The third cake was eaten by the boy when the mother was not around. We believe that a piece of mother's cake in a teenage boy's stomach can perform a positive emotional service, even if he refuses to acknowledge it.

The parents feel empowered by events like these, because their care is no longer dependent on the child's acceptance. The child, in turn, learns that their hostility does not change their parents' feelings about them.

A mother smuggled into her 16-year-old son's school bag bonbons wrapped in pieces of paper with unexpected messages of appreciation (e.g., "I know no one can defeat you!" and "I know that what you did last week was out of loyalty to your friends!"). A couple of weeks before, the boy had threatened suicide in the course of a heated argument with his mother. We believe he might have experienced the smuggled "care-bonbons" as miniature reminders of reasons to go on living.

After Alan (29) attempted suicide twice in a matter of months, his father started writing him every day. The notes were short, no more than a paragraph long. In those messages the father expressed his love, recounted stories about the past and pasted photos from their trips together. The father did this every day for months. After a year, Alan told his father that his messages had kept him alive until he was no longer in crisis.

A Detailed Case of Suicide Crisis

Martha and Eli came to therapy two months after their son Roby (21) sent them a text message from college telling them that he had failed at everything and could not go on living. They rushed to the town in which he was studying and found him drunk. At first, he rejected their offer to take him home and accused them of destroying his life. However, after some persuasion, he agreed to leave with them. In the following weeks, Roby repeatedly alluded to taking his own life. Martha became depressed and was deeply fearful whenever Roby went out. Eli felt totally paralyzed by his threats. The parents' plight was worsened by the fact that Roby refused to see a therapist or psychiatrist.

Roby would take his mother's car to go out at night, return early in the morning and stay in bed for most of the day. When he wanted to go out one night, but the car was out of gas, he berated Martha for her negligence. He complained that his parents had interfered with his decision to put an end to his life, adding that the next time he would not be so dumb as to give them notice.

The parents told the therapist that their relationship with Roby had always been stormy. When they made demands on him, Roby would silence them with a tantrum or threaten to vanish from their lives. He had had three rounds of individual therapy but without results.

The parents were asked to list the services they provided for Roby that, to their minds, were not appropriate for a 21 year old. It turned out that they had a characteristic division of labor: Eli took care of all the practical things (he had helped Roby register at the university, arranged for the dorm, made the money transfers and settled his credit card debts). Martha took charge of Roby's emotional needs, talking to him over the phone, sometimes for hours on end. The conversations, which Martha called "blaming orgies," were torture for her, but she was afraid to stop them.

With the therapist's help, the parents painted a picture of the coercive patterns between Roby and themselves. All services connected to Roby's threats or their fear of Roby's reactions were now seen as parts of a vicious cycle. The connection between inappropriate services, escalating patterns and misguided attempts to help on the one hand, and Roby's threats and overreactions on the other, became clear to the parents. Eli and Martha agreed that the goals of therapy should be to help them manifest presence, while, at the same time, they would cease giving in to Roby's demands or provocations. They were assisted in writing an announcement and were asked to compile a list of supporters.

The second session took place three days after the first. The parents and the therapist discussed how to deliver the announcement and brace themselves for Roby's reaction. Eli objected to bringing in supporters, but the fact that Roby's brothers, Martha's brothers and the two surviving grandparents knew about the suicide threats helped Eli to accept that discretion was not a viable course. A supporters' meeting was scheduled for a week later. In the meantime, the grandparents and Roby's uncles arranged to be available by phone when the announcement was made. In the announcement, Martha and Eli declared they would do all in their power to stay in touch with Roby. They stated that they would reduce their inappropriate services, for they now understood how damaging they were. They said that they were willing to help with any constructive plans but would no longer maintain his present lifestyle.

Unexpectedly, Roby remained silent and even reread the announcement after the parents delivered it orally. He remained in his room until the evening, then left the house without a word, as usual. The parents sent him a text asking when he was coming back. When Roby did not respond, they called three of his friends and asked them to tell Roby that they were extremely worried. Roby called Martha back and asked her if they had gone crazy. Martha said they would not have bothered his friends if Roby had informed them of his plans. Roby hung up angrily. The next day, his grandfather called Roby, telling him that if he disappeared, he would support the parents in looking for him, because neither he nor they were ready to give him up. He invited Roby to stay with him for a couple of days.

Twelve people attended the supporters' meeting. The supporters agreed to be on call in case Roby made a threat. A couple of close family friends who lived abroad were also included. They promised to support Roby via phone and mail. Their contribution was important, because Roby thought highly of them. A friend of Eli's, who was a financial advisor, agreed to talk to Roby about money. He made it clear to Roby that the parents would no longer rescue him if his credit card was canceled. He told Roby that he knew he was indebted to his friends and that he would be glad to help him develop a financial plan.

Over the next week, Roby threatened suicide twice. Both times, his parents called supporters, who came to the house or contacted Roby by phone. In one case, Roby was violent and two supporters took him for a long drive. They stayed with him until late at night. At about four o'clock in the morning, Roby asked to return home to sleep. One of the supporters proposed that he let things cool down with Eli and Martha by not going home right away. Instead, he would stay in the supporter's house. Roby agreed and ended up staying with this family for three days. During this time, he agreed to let the financial advisor help him plan a budget. He also accepted the supporter's suggestion that he see a psychiatrist, advice he had flatly rejected when it came from his parents. He was referred to a psychiatrist who had worked with us before. The psychiatrist told Roby that he would keep his parents apprised of the treatment but not reveal anything about his personal life. After a brief discussion of those limits, Roby agreed. The psychiatrist updated the parents and was, in turn, updated by the NVR therapist. In this way, with the help of the parents' support network, Roby became able to get professional assistance.

When Roby would start blaming Martha, she would end the conversation. On those occasions, the two supporters from abroad proved particularly helpful. They would call Roby and tell him that the blaming, besides being disrespectful to his mother, was not helping him. However, they trusted him to be able to weather the crisis. Those conversations were much shorter than the ones with Martha. Those supporters also helped smuggle in parental messages of appreciation and reminders of times when Roby had done something special. They would say, "Your father told me how you fixed the car on your trip abroad when it seemed you were stuck for the night. I didn't know about that." "Your mother told me that she could always count on you when she was in trouble.

She told me how you accompanied your younger brother to school and back for a month when he was threatened by bullies."

Roby went back to college after the semester break. Martha was sad that their special relationship had cooled; Roby now preferred to talk to Eli instead of Martha. At the final session the therapist and parents discussed how to react if the difficulties resurfaced. When Roby was in his third year of college, he had a new crisis with manic symptoms. It turned out he had been taking Ecstasy. He agreed to see the psychiatrist with whom he had built a good relationship. The psychiatrist convinced him to accept a brief hospitalization. After two weeks in the hospital, the symptoms subsided and he was discharged to his parents' home.

The parents came to a few sessions and the supporters were mobilized. Their help was vital in getting Roby to keep up with the medical treatment. Roby's problems were far from over, but the conditions for dealing with them were better than they had been in the past.

Indications and Contra-Indications for Using NVR in Situations of Suicide Threat

A possible concern regarding NVR are potential contra-indications, especially in cases of severe psychopathology. It should be stressed that in complex clinical conditions, NVR is only a part of the therapeutic process. The suicidal person and the family may require several kinds of professional attention. The fact that NVR establishes systematic connections with social and professional helpers facilitates integration among these factors.

In effect, NVR has been implemented in cases of severe psychopathology, such as hospitalized psychotic teens (Goddard et al., 2009), adolescents and adults with HFASD (Golan et al., 2018), and young adults with depression and borderline or avoidant personality disorder (Lebowitz et al., 2012).

An important concern is whether NVR could be dangerous. We believe this is possible, unless certain care measures are taken. First, NVR can be misused to challenge the child in a provocative way. Constant therapeutic attention should be devoted to this issue. Parents should be helped to communicate with the child in a supportive and never in a controlling way. In addition, it is important to assign one or more members of the helpers' group a clear role in support of the child. The best candidates for this role are those who have a positive relationship with the child. A clear offer of support strengthens the positive voices in the young person's inner parliament. In the absence of such a candidate, it might be justified to contact the child's friends. Such friends would usually not take part in the supporters' gathering, to prevent conflicts of loyalty, but they should be informed that the young person is in acute crisis and has threatened suicide. Under such conditions, friends usually become particularly good helpers.

We would like to conclude with what we view as special indications for using NVR in cases of suicide threat, compared to an approach with a wider evidence base, such as Dialectical Behavior Therapy or Attachment Based Family Therapy.

(a) NVR is indicated when threats are voiced in a clear context of intimidation.

(b) NVR is indicated when the adult-child refuses individual or family therapy.

(c) NVR is indicated when the parents feel obliged to accommodate, either because of clear threats or because they conjure up the threat of suicide in their own minds.

(d) NVR is indicated for the parents, in order to help them reduce their helplessness and suffering.

(e) NVR is indicated when the parents suffer from deep isolation, among other reasons, because of shame or the constraints imposed by the adult-child.

(f) NVR and Dialectical Behavior Therapy have different paths for preventing escalation. Given that NVR's evidence base is considerably smaller, we think that when both sides show lack of emotional regulation, especially in their mutual interactions, and the adult-child is willing to participate, Dialectical Behavior Therapy should be preferred.

(g) The reaction of most professionals to a child who mentions suicide is the desire to increase the flow of positive affection. For this reason, an approach that is purely based on improving the quality of attachment might have a more immediate appeal in this area. In effect, we think that, in many cases, the adequacy of such an approach is beyond doubt. Diamond et al. (2010; 2012) demonstrated that in cases where suicide ideation is directly linked to the absence of positive affect and to a deep sense of rejection (e.g., adolescents who are at odds with their parents because of their sexual orientation), focusing treatment on improving parental acceptance and the quality of the parent–child bond not only improves the relationship but also reduces depression and suicidality. We see a continuum between cases in which suicide ideation arises from a sense of neglect and rejection and cases in which suicide threats emerge in the context of demands for inappropriate services. Ideally, one should be able to match the treatment to the child's position on that continuum. Families closer to the neglect–rejection pole would then receive Attachment Based Family Therapy, while families closer to the escalation–coercion end would receive an NVR intervention. But we want to stress that NVR aims at restoring and stabilizing the parent–child bond. In this respect, it is not only not opposed to Attachment Based Family Therapy but can clearly be viewed as attachment-oriented. In effect, NVR has been proposed as a bridge between parental authority and secure attachment through the provision of a parental anchor (Omer et al., 2013).

5   Helping Parents of Children and Adolescents at Risk of Failure to Emerge*

In Chapter 1, we characterized adult-children as people who at some point stop progressing toward psychosocial adulthood. Our encounters with their families have shown that this progression can halt during adolescence. The main problematic behaviors we identified as possible precursors of entrenched dependence were: (a) digital abuse; (b) school avoidance and social withdrawal; (c) tyrannical attitudes; and (d) irresponsible financial behavior.

Research on adolescents and adults who withdrew from social life to the extent of showing clearly reduced ability to function in the external world points to a probable continuity between these two populations. In a much quoted study, a large group of adolescents, who displayed similar characteristics to many adult-children, were categorized as being at "invisible risk" for suicide (Carli et al., 2014). Although the youth in this group were low on "visible" risk factors such as illegal drug use and excessive alcohol consumption, they exhibited high media use, sedentary behavior and reduced sleep. It turned out that these socially withdrawn, digitally addicted and sleepless young people were suffering from similar levels of suicidal ideation, anxiety and depression as their peers at "visible" risk. We believe that adolescents at invisible risk have a greater chance of becoming dysfunctional adult-children.

Two factors may be colluding to obscure this continuity: First, many of these youngsters are able to maintain a veneer of normative behavior that prevents detection of their highly problematic condition; and second, in most countries there are still strict transitional divisions between mental health services for children and for adults. The dividing line falls at the age of 18. Presumably professionals who treat children and adolescents hardly ever see adults in their practice and vice versa. Even academic journals make this distinction, thus contributing to the selective blindness that prevented bringing the phenomenon to light. As we mentioned, when our work with the parents of dysfunctional children and adolescents became known, more and more parents of adults started coming to us. A trickle became a flood. Our position in the professional field has thus allowed us to witness this continuity with special clarity.

---

* The section on Digital Abuse was coauthored by Yaron Sela and Merav Zach.

More research is needed to clarify the developmental pathways leading from invisible risk or social withdrawal in adolescence to entrenched dependence in adulthood, as well as more interdisciplinary collaboration across the line between pre- and post-18 healthcare. In the meantime, this chapter proposes ways in which parents of adolescents can identify the early patterns that might be predictors of AED, thus reducing immediate damage and developmental risk.

Digital Abuse

This term applies to all forms of dependence on screens in any format. The smartphone might be said to be another family member in many households. It is present in almost every encounter between children and their friends or parents, but with different roles. When children are with their peers, the smartphone is social glue. One of us (Haim Omer) recently travelled on a train full of teenagers who had gotten out of school, all of whom were sitting together, talking to each other and holding smartphones. Some were speaking with one another and others showing their friends what was on their screens. It was evident that the device contributed to the communication and helped fill up dead moments, providing content for further communication. The children did not get lost in their smartphones but used them to create a common reality. This is not how they use their smartphones when they are with their parents. All it takes is a quick glance at families in restaurants. In this context, the smartphone almost always separates and isolates: children are absorbed in their phones, far from their parents' worlds.

Parents feel a particular helplessness when it comes to the virtual world, among other reasons, because of their sense of technological inferiority. The relationship between parents and children in the virtual realm has been likened to that between immigrants and natives. For many parents this world is foreign; they look at it from the outside and feel awkward there, unlike their children. Given this gap, many parents give up. This leaves the child alone facing the dangers of the virtual world.

Given the difficulties and the extent of their helplessness, many parents would be surprised that it may take only a short time to reduce their sense of alienation and the risks to which their children are exposed. In a study of parents who were worried about their children's digital activities, we found that after three sessions of group training, parents stopped feeling helpless, increased their presence and reduced harmful practices (Sela, 2019). We showed that the parents knew more, were more willing to undertake protective steps and succeeded in reducing the number of hours the child spent in front of the screen, especially late at night. This is the first study in which smartphone abuse was objectively measured through data provided by the server, and not only by subjective report. We believe that increasing parents' presence in their children's digital world at least through adolescence is the best guarantee against the development of digital abuse that characterizes dysfunctional dependence in adulthood (Omer, 2017). The following are some of the issues that parents can learn to confront.

Coping with Digital Abuse

The child's pernicious absorption can be manifested by increasing disengagement from the familial and social environment, a decline in academic achievement, increased seclusion, sleep disturbance or even complete abandonment of functioning in the real world in favor of the virtual one.

Many parents ask whether, how much and how to restrict the use of screens. Experience shows that limiting the number of hours per day is often ineffective. Such restriction may put the parents in the role of inspectors who count the hours and argue with the child. This atmosphere harms the relationship and exhausts the parents. Rather than setting a designated number of hours, parents can stipulate a few clear-cut rules such as, "No smartphones before leaving for school, during meals or after 10 p.m." The advantage of these rules is that they are less amenable to bargaining.

Parents should not think they can maintain those limits without serious preparation. The attempt to impose limits on screen use by demands and threats is doomed to fail. The world of screens has such sweeping presence in the child's life that the parents' protests tend to vanish. The situation changes if the parents approach the task with the patience and seriousness it requires. To do so, they should coordinate their positions, announce their limits unequivocally (preferably by a formal announcement), build support and legitimacy for their position, and prepare for decisive action if the limits are violated.

Benny and Gloria attended a lecture on problematic screen use. They consulted the speaker on how to change their children's habit of staring at their smartphones during meals, which had become an unpleasant routine. The parents prepared a written announcement, gathered their three children (aged 15, 14 and 10) around the table, and told them:

Recently our meals have stopped being family occasions. Instead, we are like a collection of separate people absorbed in their smartphones. We decided that we are going to do whatever is needed to change this situation, which is very damaging to our family spirit. Dad and I have decided to turn off our phones during meals. This rule will apply to you as well. There will be no more smartphones at table. We are going to demand that you turn your smartphones off so that there will be no rings during meals. We have shared this decision with your grandparents, your two aunts and their children, so that when we have a meal at our house everyone will have to turn off their phones.

At the next meal, the parents turned off their phones in their children's presence and asked them to do the same. Nobody objected. The parents asked their relatives to respect the same rule when they came to visit. The ritual of turning off the phones also took place at the grandparents' home, thus reinforcing the rule. Gloria's younger sister was impressed and adopted the same rule for her family. Benny's sister did not feel the need for a similar restriction in her home but agreed to respect the rule every time she and her children had dinner at Benny and Gloria's.

When the parents detect signals that indicate their child is using the smartphone or computer in damaging ways, they must take stronger preventing measures. Here are some typical warning signs that justify a more determined intervention:

- Locking the door when on the computer.
- Sitting in front of a screen until late at night.
- Making unauthorized charges on the parents' credit card.
- Neglecting school in favor of virtual activities.
- Avoiding meals and other family activities.
- Withdrawing from social activities.
- Screaming at the parents when interrupted on the computer.

The best way to begin the process of resistance is by a formal announcement. What follows is a possible text:

We know how important the computer is in your life. But we have noticed that your use of the computer harms your functioning in basic areas like school and sleep. We will do whatever we can to stop it and make sure you use your computer in constructive and not destructive ways.

After the announcement comes the implementation. The following are some recommended practical steps.

Setting a Time When All Screens Are Turned Off   The parents must set a time after which all screens are to be shut down. It is recommended that the parents should not turn the computer off while the child is using it. This often leads to escalation. There are several ways to move forward without falling into that trap, such as telling the child that, if they do not turn off the computer, the parents will disable it. The parents should then disable the computer when the child is not present, for instance by removing a modem or a mouse. Another way is to tell the child, "You have five minutes to save your work and turn the computer off. Afterwards we'll make sure it is shut down." If the child does not comply, the parents should cut off the electricity for a few seconds. Doing so from a safe distance reduces the violent potential of pressing the off button. A supporter can warn the child that the parents are going to turn off the electricity. If the parents expect the child to react violently, they should shut down the computer the next day and leave it disabled until the child commits to following the rules. Involving supporters is crucial for preventing escalation and legitimizing the parents' position. In addition, the child's commitment in the presence of witnesses is usually more binding than a commitment made only before the parents.

Cutting Off Internet Service   Sometimes, online connectivity needs to be shut down for a while. This requires parental commitment and preparation. The child also uses the Internet for necessary activities such as downloading homework from the school website. The parents should make alternative arrangements to allow for school work for the duration of the internet shutdown. One possibility of which many parents are not aware is ordering internet services only at designated hours. There are also smartphone apps that shut it off at a predetermined hour every day. Children who are used to spending days and nights in front of the computer may protest when they lose internet access. However, our experience with hundreds of families shows that most parents can cut off internet connectivity or shut off the smartphone if they prepare themselves and rally supporters. In our experience, the nightmare scenarios that many parents fear do not materialize. Shutting down screens may be met with fury or tears, but the readiness of parents to act in planned and determined ways ultimately empowers them and lowers the risks involved in children's problematic online exposure.

Confiscating the Smartphone   This measure evokes intense anxiety in many parents. Many view the smartphone as almost a natural extension of the child and its confiscation as the violation of a sacred taboo. Parents are also afraid of what might happen if they were unable to contact their child when away from home. These concerns should be addressed when the parents prepare to take the child's smartphone. In most of our cases, the confiscation was only for a few days, and in a handful of cases a few weeks.

Some teenagers rebelled by using their own money to buy new smartphones. In those cases, the parents forbade the child from using the smartphone in their home. Parents understand that such a measure is justified when the phone is likened to an addictive drug. Just as they would not let their child consume illicit drugs in their home, they should not allow them to be addicted to screens in their home. But under no circumstances should there be a scuffle over the smartphone. Some parents inform their child that if they used the smartphone at home, in spite of their prohibition, they would take it away. Later, the parents removed it while the child was sleeping, or demanded that the child turn it over in the presence of supporters. The supporters help not only by backing the parental measure but also by helping the child get the phone back once the required restrictions have been accepted. Parents are often surprised that their child accepts the new regulations, when the proposal is presented in a respectful way by a third party.

Simon and René watched helplessly as their daughter Rhea (16) dropped out of school, spending days and nights on Facebook. When their therapist suggested that they limit her use of the smartphone, Simon cried, "That is an extreme approach. It's as if you asked me to cut off my daughter's arm! How do I know it won't lead to depression or her doing something drastic?" Later in the conversation, it became clear that Rhea had never threatened to harm herself and was not depressed. The therapist explained that even had there been such threats, the response would not be to maintain the sanctity of Rhea's virtual world at the expense of normal functioning. The therapist focused on the phrase "cut off my daughter's arm," which expressed the exaggerated fear and sense of illegitimacy of any action related to the smartphone. After a process in which the parents prepared for different scenarios of resistance by their daughter, they made an announcement, intensified their supervision and, when none of this led to improvement, disconnected the computer and took away her smartphone.

To their surprise, when this happened, Rhea finished protesting. Once she saw that her parents had made good on their promise, she immediately began negotiating. The discussions lasted more than two weeks. All through this time, Rhea managed to live without her computer or smartphone. The reason it took so long was that the parents demanded that Rhea resume her studies. There were still some difficulties after the computer and smartphone were restored, but Rhea's functional impairment was considerably reduced. When at the end of the process the therapist mentioned the father's fear he was about to cut off his daughter's arm, Simon said: "I can't believe I thought that. As if the smartphone were as sacred as my daughter's life!"

Abed and Nida were the parents of Mark (14), who until the previous year had been an excellent student, active in the Boy Scouts and popular. Nothing prepared his parents for the change that came when he started playing online games. Within a few months, Mark withdrew from almost all social activity and his academic performance declined steeply. He started coming home late and leaving early, to sit in the park for a couple of hours and play the game on his smartphone. His relationship with his parents, which had previously been close, rapidly worsened.

The parents prepared an announcement, which they delivered to Mark in the presence of two grandparents, an uncle, an aunt and an older cousin, Roy, whom Mark admired. In the announcement, the parents said they would do everything they could to resist the gaming addiction that was taking over Mark's life. After the meeting, Roy invited Mark for a meeting to discuss possibilities for a dignified resolution. They met in a café. After a two-hour discussion, they wrote a joint proposal. Mark promised not to turn on the game before finishing his schoolwork for that day. He also agreed not to turn on the computer until after dinner and only in the presence of one parent or one of the supporters, whose job it was to log the time when Mark began playing and warn him 15 minutes before his allotted three hours were up. He committed to turning off the computer when he got that message. Mark also promised not to play the game on his smartphone and that, if he broke his promise, he would lose the smartphone, as well as the right to have a computer in his room. Roy agreed with Mark on a plan of how to make up for his missed schoolwork. Within two months, Mark had made good on the areas of his life that he had neglected. The big surprise was that Mark came to the conclusion that the game was ruining his life. Within a short time, the agreement on the terms of computer use became moot, because Mark stopped playing the game completely.

Parents often complain that none of these steps can guarantee that the child will not continue their pernicious computer use elsewhere or in other ways. This objection helps us clarify to the parents the deeper meaning of NVR. The parents can resist harmful use but they cannot determine what the child will do. Resistance is meaningful, even when the child succeeds in circumventing it. The message the parents convey is, "We will not supply you with the means to destroy yourself." Or, "We will not agree that our home become a shelter of stagnation." The fact that the child succeeds in getting what they want outside, or sometimes in cheating the parents within the house, does not invalidate their resistance.

The similarity between this work with the parents of adolescents and our treatment protocol for the parents of adult-children is obvious. By acting decisively to disrupt the child's abuse of screens, the parents are performing important preventive work against AED. We explain this to the parents: "Your child's computer abuse puts their future at risk. They may be the kind of adolescent that becomes more and more withdrawn and addicted to screens, to the point where they become incapable of functioning in real life." This inspires many parents to act. We are only saying openly what they have already surmised.

School Refusal and Social Withdrawal

Many adult-children have a history of school refusal and social withdrawal. School refusal often appears in early to middle childhood, and becomes chronic in adolescence. Dropout may also occur during high school or college. The precipitating event may be scholastic failure, an acute mental crisis or failure in adjusting to life away from the parental home. Social withdrawal in adolescence often continues into adulthood. The youth may then withdraw into the home or even into their own room.

School refusal has vast repercussions on the child's identity. The role of student includes not only scholastic performance but also a definition of daily routine, a sense of belonging, a reference group and a future orientation. As school refusal becomes chronic, the child's identity as a student is replaced by harmful forms of self-characterization, such as "incapable," "weird" or "sick." The child's inner dialogue becomes characterized by defeatist beliefs such as, "I can't stand the pressure!" "I don't belong!" "I am a failure!" These beliefs are unwittingly reinforced by the surroundings, for instance by a psychiatric label, a reduction in functional expectations and the creation of an artificial environment that fosters passivity.

Most parents waver between pressuring the child to go back to school by threats and punishments, or identifying with the child's suffering and allowing them to stay at home. Often both approaches fail, leaving the parents and the child helpless.

Our program for school refusal (Omer et al., 2016) is designed to help parents function as an anchor that resists the forces driving the child away from school and threatening their identity as a student. The process aims to help parents restore their guiding role and recover their effaced presence.

As in our program with the parents of adult-children, work with parents of school-avoidant children includes an announcement, the development of a support network (in which the teachers play a central role), a plan for reducing parental accommodation and proactive steps for maintaining the child's identity as a student. Parents and teachers develop a plan together for keeping the child informed on curriculum, homework and school events. Contact with classmates and teachers is maintained or renewed. It is important to preserve a regular school day schedule, even if the child is staying home. The parents make sure that the school bag is packed the night before. Extracurricular activities that conflict with school attendance or reinforce absenteeism are prohibited. A plan for transitioning back to school is developed, preferably in cooperation with the child. Supporters from the school and the extended family help the child cope with academic difficulties or problems with teachers or classmates.

Despite the many similarities with our program for the parents of adult-children, there is also an important difference. Parents of school-age children are responsible for their child's attendance; adult-children are, at least legally, responsible for themselves. Therefore it is not the job of parents of adult-children to get the adult-child ready to fulfil their commitments, accompany them to work or consult with college professors in the search of solutions to the problems that may be keeping them away from attending classes. Parents of adult-children should limit themselves to launching their child into the world outside; they do not have to escort them there.

Even parents of younger children have clear limitations on their responsibility for the child's dysfunction. Thus, the parents of an adolescent with social withdrawal should not invite the child's friends over, make phone calls that their anxious child avoids making, or mediate between the child and the external world. The parents can encourage the child's social contacts but should not accommodate the child's avoidance by doing things for them. Stopping accommodation and preventing the formation of a degenerative shelter are clear roles for the parents of a socially anxious child. Persuading, nagging or badgering an adolescent to become socially involved often backfires. Parental resistance is usually far more important than parental push. Preaching, threats or bribery are always inappropriate.

All the means that we have described for stopping accommodation and dismantling the degenerative shelter are relevant for children with school refusal and social withdrawal. With some adolescents, the level of parental engagement and resistance must be as high as for adult-children. Therefore, parents who learn to conduct a determined but nonescalating struggle with a recalcitrant adolescent will be in a good position to prevent the formation of a full-fledged dysfunctional bond. They will recognize the signs and avoid the typical errors of the parents of adult-children. Parents whom we treated when their child was an adolescent sometimes come back to us when there is a relapse in early adulthood. It turns out that those parents are better prepared to cope with the crisis than parents who came to us first when their child was already an adult.

Children with "Tyrannical Behaviors"

Another precursor of Adult Entrenched Dependence is the development of severe controlling and domineering attitudes during childhood and adolescence. Those behaviors signify a steep inversion of the usual family hierarchy, to the point that those children have been described as "tyrannical" (Franc & Omer, 2017). Those patterns may appear very early (in some cases with three-year-old children). The diagnoses that have been associated with those children include separation or social anxiety, oppositional-defiant, OCD, HFASD and emotional dysregulation disorders. Common to all is the children's tendency to impose their will by screams, tantrums, extreme threats and physical attacks, or in more subtle ways, such as exploiting their medical condition, having panic attacks or implying that they will harm themselves when the parents do not comply. The following points may help clarify if a child has tyrannical behaviors.

Are You Afraid of Your Child's Reactions?

This is a subjective criterion that is not necessarily related to the child's actual behaviors or age. Thus, some parents of very young children live in abject terror of their tantrums. Understanding the parents' fears may help overcome them. For example, some parents don't dare upset a child with a physical illness, so as not to cause them additional pain. Some of those children may exaggerate their health issues, in order to control their parents. This may be the case with many children with blue spells or childhood diabetes. Usually, the controlling child uses a variety of means to frighten the parents. Thus, a diabetic child may play on the parents' fears of a glycemic hypo or get lost every now and then to keep them on edge (Rothmann-Kabir, 2018).

Have You Renounced Important Activities Because of Your Child's Problems?

Most parents will at some point relinquish some of their own activities to accommodate a difficult child, but in families with this problem, parents tend to sacrifice basic functions. Thus, some divorced parents give up their right to a relationship with a new partner because the child insists, "It's either me or your spouse!" Some interrupt their professional careers. Others limit their social life, either because of restrictions imposed by the child or because they feel they are disbelieved or criticized by others. Those criticisms are a common experience, as many of those children behave infinitely better outside than inside their home, leading even close relations to question the parents' reports or blame them for their troubles.

Are You Hindered by Your Child in Routine Decisions?

In some families, the child controls the food that is served, who sits where at the table or which family member gets to take the first shower in the morning. Siblings are obliged to comply, otherwise they risk sanctions from the controlling child or complaints from the parents, who count on their understanding to keep the peace. Many siblings of a domineering child never forgive their parents for having sacrificed their well-being to the needs of their problematic brother or sister.

Are You Ashamed of What Is Happening at Home?

Shame is closely related to isolation. Many parents tell us that the situation at home is so bizarre that they refrain from describing it to others. Shame also affects their self-image as parents. They go about thinking that they have failed in a basic task. Dealing with the parents' shame is a central task in preparing them to meet with supporters. Getting to know other parents with similar problems can be of great help. This is one of the advantages of the NVR group treatment for parents of children with tyrannical behaviors that we developed with our colleagues in France (Franc & Omer, 2017).

Is Your Child Violent?

It is important that the therapist diligently addresses the issue of violence, because parents tend to minimize it. For instance, a mother in our treatment once said that when her 15-year-old son became upset, he would start moving his hands and feet. It took some questioning to unearth the fact that her son's hands and feet did not just "move around," but that she had been beaten black and blue several times. Also, verbal violence requires detailed description. Thus, a child who yells "Shut up!" cannot be compared to a child who hurls deep insults at their parents. One type of violence that we have witnessed almost exclusively in those families manifests itself in clinging physically to the parent, yelling directly into their ear or coming into their room at night to prevent them from sleeping. The message of this kind of violence is very different from that of a child with conduct disorder. Whereas the latter may hit the parents to get them out of the way, the tyrannical child behaves in ways that say, "You belong to me!" This message of possession is emblematic of this type of relationship.

Although the relationship between those children and their parents is often similar to the oppressive bond we have described between parents and adult-children, there is one important difference. With few exceptions, adult-children want to be left alone. They are already sure that the parents cannot escape, so they are not interested in controlling the parents' every move. However, if the parents take steps to stop their services, some typical behaviors of "tyrannical children" may reappear.

Our program for the parents of tyrannical children has many parallels to the treatment we described in Chapter 3. Those parents have to learn about the nefarious effects of accommodation, the differences between dysfunctional and functional dependence, the process of escalation, the announcement, the support network and the process of de-accommodation. The parents of "tyrannical children" who succeed in this task may be preventing the development of AED.

Irresponsible Financial Behavior

Adolescents who are financially irresponsible develop a different kind of dependence than those whose behavior is characterized by internet abuse, school refusal, social withdrawal or extreme controlling behaviors. They often live away from the parental home but remain dependent in ways that are no less destructive than adult-children who remain bound to it. They often display a brazen entitlement, behaving as if the parents' obligation to cover their debts, reckless spending, traffic tickets or gambling were self-evident. If parents show signs of reluctance, they may react like other adult-children, or threaten to go to loan sharks.

The parents of adolescents with these behavior patterns can help their children by openly discussing financial issues with them. Money is a good subject to discuss, since parents can use simple arithmetic to support their arguments. If the child's explanations do not add up, there are surely some omissions or discrepancies in the child's reports. Financial behavior is thus well-suited for creating transparency. However, many parents avoid a pointed discussion, even though they see the writing on the wall.

When I (Haim Omer) was 15, I started working at my parents' tobacco shop in Sao Paulo, which was managed by Abraham, my mother's cousin. I used to take over his shift every day at noon for two hours. According to the agreement, I received 50 cruzeiros a day for my work. I took the money directly from the till. Abraham loved me and we had a close and equal relationship that went far beyond what might be expected in light of the age gap between us. This might have contributed to his turning a blind eye to the fact that I didn't just settle for the agreed sum, but took some added compensation, both in the form of cigarettes and additional sums that I allowed myself without reporting. I tricked myself into believing that my thefts were going unnoticed. My parents never asked questions, trusting that Abraham would keep an eye on me. Only two years after I had started working at the store, Abraham shattered my illusion, when he gave me a strong hint that he knew exactly how much money was missing from the till. I was ashamed and stopped stealing cash (though I kept stocking up on cigarettes). Throughout the years, I wondered how his forgiving disregard might have affected my life. I believe it added to my undisciplined attitude toward money, which characterized my financial behavior as a young adult.

In addition, there were serious pitfalls into which I had almost fallen. I had a friend 10 years older than me who got into trouble with debt, and embezzled money from the travel agency where he worked. He told me of a tricky ploy by which he thought he could more than repay his debts. He asked me to help him with a sum of money that he needed in order to execute his scheme. Fortunately, this occurred right after Abraham had made it clear to me that he knew about the missing money. If it hadn't been for that, I might well have agreed to help my friend get out of his mess and got into a mess of my own.

A good way to start the conversation about money is to tell the child, "We know you're getting into financial trouble. We want to talk to you so as best to help you stop whatever is leading you into this trouble." Such a message shows that the parents are acting out of love and concern. A major goal of the conversation is to engender transparency. This is true not only with children and adolescents, but also with an adult-child with debts who expects to be rescued by their parents.

When Kaylin (15) was a young child, his parents opened a savings accounts for him. Kaylin pressured his parents into handing him direct access to his savings and promptly spent most of them on his stamp collection. Later, he developed a passion for electronic gadgets, sold his stamp collection, and started to buy and sell gadgets online. Then the parents found out that he was gambling. He had sold all his electronic devices and spent the income on sports bets. He began neglecting his studies and borrowed additional gambling funds from his friends. Two months after the parents found out about the gambling and the debts, Kaylin's grandmother reported to them that he had come to her in tears, begging for money to repay a friend. He promised it would never happen again and made her promise that she would not tell them. The grandmother gave him the money and kept the secret, but when the parents told her about Kaylin's gambling, she told them about what had happened. The parents told Kaylin that they knew about the debts, the gambling and the money he had taken from his grandmother. They told him they were going to keep a close eye on him. Kaylin, his father and his brother went together to the convenience stores that sold Kaylin his gambling forms. The sellers promised not to sell him any more forms. The father also contacted some of Kaylin's friends and told them his son was at great risk of becoming addicted to gambling. Most of the friends responded positively and told the father they would not cooperate with Kaylin's purchasing of gambling forms or any other gambling activities. The parents gathered the extended family, explained the problem to them and asked everyone to refuse Kaylin's requests for money. It turned out he had already managed to get money from his other grandmother and solicited loans from two older cousins. The parents announced to Kaylin they would make periodic checks in his room. The situation appeared to calm down. Two years later, however, they found a gambling form in his room. At that point they confronted Kaylin and reinstated the close supervision. The parents now knew that Kaylin was at serious risk of becoming addicted to gambling. Though they had succeeded in getting him reasonably clean until the end of high school, they were not at all sure about what the future would bring. At least, no untoward developments would catch them off guard.

The following case illustrates how transparency was achieved with an adult-child who refused to disclose his financial situation while expecting his debts to be paid by the parents.

Roy (27) was financially dependent on his parents. He lived in an apartment they rented for him and they paid all his expenses. In the past, Roy had shown himself able to keep a job. However, he had dreamt of becoming an actor and his parents allowed him to pursue his dream. He was admitted into a reputable school but dropped out during the first year. He applied for another acting school but did not pass the auditions. After this, he did not return to work and his parents continued to provide him the same monthly sum as when he was studying, partly because they viewed him as a person with an artistic bent. However, he seemed to be needing more money than they were giving him. He turned to his parents for more financial help after his bank notified him that his credit card was about to be blocked. The parents decided they had to achieve full transparency with him, but Roy refused to disclose his accounts, arguing that they were his private business. The parents told him they were willing to consult a professional, who would go through his accounts with him and help him prepare a financial plan. They told him they were willing to help him get out of debt but only under professional supervision. The financial counselor would provide the parents with summarized reports that would not specify the details of Roy's expenses. He agreed to the parents' terms and collaborated with the financial counselor.

A year later, he had paid off most of his debts and paid back some of the money that his parents had given him to keep him afloat. After a couple of stable years, the parents were tempted to give Roy a gift for his 30th birthday, allowing him to fulfill his dream of a theater trip to London. To their astonishment, the trip to London ended with new debts, threatening to destroy Roy's hard-won stability. The parents rehired the financial counselor. The event made it clear that they had to be careful of any situation where Roy could enjoy their financial services in an unsupervised way.

6   Addressing Entrenched Dependence in Special Contexts

The intervention manual that we presented in Chapter 3 requires adaptation to the particular conditions in which the family comes for help. The situation differs, for instance, if parents present an acute emergency or a chronic situation, if the adult-child is concurrently in psychiatric inpatient care or refuses to leave their room, or if the parents are in their 60s or older. In this chapter, we will describe how to adapt the intervention, utilizing the peculiarities of each situation as potential levers for change.

Emergencies

Often parents come to us when they have experienced an emergency, such as a violent outburst, attempted suicide, psychotic breakdown or trouble with the police. Each family defines crisis in its own terms. For many parents, it is when an adolescent moves from verbal to physical violence, or from suicide threats to an actual attempt. Emergencies offer opportunities, for an extraordinary event justifies extraordinary measures. In emergencies, the tasks that are part of the intervention's early stages can be expedited. Often, the announcement and supporters' gathering can take place in a few days. Emergencies justify breaking taboos and crossing lines that had never been crossed before. The alert therapist who seizes the opportunity may find that a strong therapeutic alliance can be established as early as the first session. In contrast, the therapist who reacts to the parents' sense of urgency at a more deliberate psychotherapeutic pace may find that the opportunity has been lost.

Coping with an emergency gives the parents a sense of empowerment. Successful crisis management, however, differs from trying to dial things down. Calming a crisis is far from empowering, for instance if the emergency resulted in additional accommodation. Our practice is the exact contrary: to leverage the emergency as an opportunity to reduce accommodation. Emergency management may thus become a model for the entire intervention.

Susan (65) was the widowed mother of two well-functioning daughters and a son, Fred (38), with a marked sense of entitlement. Fred lived in an apartment that Susan owned, worked only occasionally and was financially indebted to many people. He would often use suicide threats to extract funds from his mother, or hint that he was being threatened by his creditors. Susan's own financial situation became increasingly tenuous, while Fred's debts did not seem to diminish.

The emergency arose when Fred started harassing his mother over the phone, insisting that she give him money and telling her he was in imminent danger. He once came to her apartment in the middle of the night, threatening that if she did not help him, she would be "responsible for the consequences." Whenever he saw her, he would chain-smoke, something he did not do anywhere else. In one of those bouts, Fred seemed to have given himself nicotine poisoning and Susan had to call for an ambulance. Susan thought he was having a heart attack.

In the course of a therapy session, she began crying and asked the therapist, "Is there any way I can get him to stop smoking?" Susan could not sleep, lost her will to live and stopped visiting her grandchildren. Her blood pressure rose and she felt pressure in her chest. She felt guilty for depriving her daughters of their father's inheritance by giving all the money to her son.

A guiding principle when dealing with an emergency is to prioritize, defining immediate and attainable goals. Susan had set herself three unattainable goals: to get Fred to stop smoking; to cover his debts; and to make him financially responsible. However, the emergency was not only Fred's, but also Susan's. This perspective allowed for the definition of different goals. Susan could be helped to resist Fred's blackmail, protect her own health, stop being available to Fred on demand and spend more time with her grandchildren. To achieve these goals, Susan had to rely on her support network. Given the intense pressure she was under, Susan was perfectly willing to enlist the help of her daughters, sons-in-law, brothers, sister and best friend.

With the supporters' help, Fred was told that his mother would no longer accept his phone calls. He could still send her messages through the supporters. He was told that his mother would be sleeping in her daughters' homes. Fred's uncle told him that, if he wanted, he would assist him in getting help from a financial consultant. With the help of her son-in-law who was a physician, Susan developed a plan for healthier living. She started taking daily walks. Her blood pressure dropped and stabilized. Her sleep improved. The time she spent with her grandchildren made her feel that she was benefitting them, her daughters and herself. It took about three weeks for Fred's pressure to abate.

Susan's change of heart became evident when, a few months later, she asked the therapist whether it would be a right decision on her part to bequeath her property to her three children in equal parts. In the past, she had been afraid of taking this step, because Fred seemed to assume that he would inherit more than his equal share, including the apartment he was living in.

Most of our cases go through acute and stable phases. Families with an adult-child often present with a steady dysfunctional condition that is punctuated by occasional crises. When the situation is stable, it may be more difficult to inspire parents to immediate action. However, the therapist should not simply wait for an emergency. Helping parents write an announcement, gather a support network and reduce accommodation are steps that may set off a controlled crisis. Such intervention-initiated crises may be particularly effective in mobilizing the parents because they can prepare in advance, rather than being caught unawares. By preparing, they become better able to control themselves, avoid escalation, rally support and build their resilience.

Worrisome Conditions

Many cases that eventually deteriorate into full-fledged AED arise out of a stressful life-event such as a breakup, the loss of a job, the death of a loved one or a road accident. Those crises, however painful, may resolve on their own with time and support. In other cases, the setback impacts various functional aspects. The young person may then take refuge in the parental home. The parents naturally want to support their suffering child. However, they must be careful not to turn the temporary resting place into a degenerative shelter. Risks are particularly high when the parents view their child as especially vulnerable, underrate their coping capacity and enable avoidance behaviors. This overlap between crisis and accommodation may prove malignant. The therapist's job is to help parents remain vigilant to harmful processes, develop a stance of support but not overprotection, formulate messages of functional expectation and develop a clear plan to prevent the situation from becoming chronic.

Concerns are a natural part of parenting and are as varied as parenting itself. The way in which parents talk about their concerns and their child tells much about their fears and desires. The parents' worries may also open a window into the past and tell us why they think this particular child got trapped in such a predicament and why they worry about this child more than they do about their other children. The therapist's questions may direct the parents' attention to the issue of accommodation, for instance: "Are you sometimes worried that perhaps you worry too much?" "Is it possible that your worrying may not be to your child's advantage?" "Do you sometimes feel that you don't relate to this child as you would to someone else his age?" "Are there things that you do out of worry for your daughter that might make her less able to cope on her own?" If these questions are asked in the right tone, the parents may feel that the therapist has touched the very heart of their parenting.

In order to evaluate the functioning potential, it is important to inquire about the child's daily routine; performance at school or work; social standing and activities; ability to perform age-appropriate tasks; and relationship to other family members. When the present picture does not clearly show that the young person has become dysfunctional, the therapist can develop some scripts with the parents that will help them reach a conclusion, if new facts arise. In such cases, the initial therapeutic contact will serve a preparatory goal, that of making the parents more alert and prepared for problematic developments.

Sam (21) was in his second year of college. His parents, Alfred and Hilda, came to us because they felt very worried that something bad was going on but were completely in the dark about his real situation. The therapist helped them to articulate their concerns and formulate some pointed questions they could pose to Sam. They came back from their meeting with Sam with the sense that he had been too eager to dispel their worries, but nevertheless there was little more they could do at the time. Thereupon, the therapist helped the parents define the thresholds and contingencies that would indicate a need to return for additional consultation.

Three weeks later, the parents found out that Sam was lying to them. He had told them he was still in college, while in fact having dropped out almost a year before. They returned to therapy and within a few sessions felt sufficiently empowered to change the terms under which they were willing to continue supporting him. They stopped providing Sam his student allowance and Sam started working temporary jobs. Two years later, they agreed to help him return to college but this time kept a close eye on what was going on with him.

Joanna (25) came back to the parental home after breaking up with her fiancé. The parents, Tino and Kim, came to us because they were worried about her mental state. She seemed depressed, and neglected her appearance. However, she went on with her job and continued to see her friends. With the therapist's help, the parents developed some scripts regarding possible changes in her mood, behavior or life situation.

The parents returned a few months later, when Joanna quit her job and started spending most of her time in her room. The therapist helped them to recruit supporters, one of whom persuaded Joanna to meet with a psychiatrist. She began taking antidepressants and after a while went back to working and socializing. Half a year later, the parents helped her to rent her own apartment.

These vignettes illustrate the course of a short preventive intervention, to help ward off possible deterioration. The therapist's ability to empathically address the parents' worries and help them develop a script regarding possible developments assisted in establishing a therapeutic alliance that proved helpful when the worrisome signs became alarming.

Preventive interventions for worrisome conditions that do not yet constitute full-fledged AED follow a common principle: The developmental time arrow is irreversible. The parents' duty is to support their child but never in a direction that goes against the course of growth. In this way, their giving serves a launching function. The parents' messages should make it clear that they will not accept a reversal of the developmental time arrow. For instance, "Are you dropping out of school? Either go to another school or start working.

Staying at home is not an option." Or, "You're in an emotional crisis and can't study or work? Let's see how you can get help to cope with your crisis. Refusing help and playing computer games is not an option." Or, "You need a period of rest at home after a bad experience outside? We're happy to see you and help you but on terms that are different from when you were a child. Just staying here and doing nothing is not an option." Launching is the process of making good on these words.

Aged Parents

A special condition that poses powerful challenges is that of frail elderly people, who are too physically weak to play the strong leading role that the NVR program customarily assigns to parents. With advanced age, the supportive pattern is often reversed, as parents may come to depend on their children because of their physical or mental condition. Often, the very fact that the adult-child is the one who is at home may give them a central role in this process. Occasionally, the reversal works to everybody's advantage. The adult-child may then be in a position to give back some of the many services they received. The parents may then gain some restitution for their years of sacrifice and hardship.

However, in many cases the picture is bleaker. Social workers who specialize in geriatric care have many heartbreaking stories to share about negligent or abusive adult-children. As the parents' mobility deteriorates, more space in the house may be claimed as the adult-child's absolute domain. We have seen cases in which an adult-child used the parent' home for drinking or gambling sprees, while a debilitated parent was left alone confined to their room. We do not presume to have a general solution for the serious social problem of elderly abuse by adult-children. However, when a working alliance can be developed with the aged parents' other children or close relatives, some remedial steps can be undertaken.

In some of our cases, a coalition of concerned children or grandchildren asked the aged parents to consent to the creation of a protective buffer between themselves and the adult-child. Sometimes social services or the police became involved, interrupting a pattern of abuse and allowing the parents to receive better care. In some of our cases, when the parents, out of a lifelong habit of protecting the adult-child, balked at authorizing their concerned children to act, the children wrote their own announcement to their vulnerable parent, and then delivered it in the presence of the support group. An 89-year-old widower received such an announcement from three of his children, with the support of six other family members:

Dear Father,

We've all come to the conclusion that you have become a prisoner in your own home. You and Mom were always willing to sacrifice yourselves for your children, especially for Johnny, on account of his mental illness. But we all think that things have gone too far. It is not right that your home, which you and Mom always loved to keep clean and orderly, should become the shelter for dozens of stray cats that turn it into a garbage pile. In the past, Johnny always fed cats in the streets without bringing them into the house. Now that you've become too weak to protest, those boundaries have been erased. This is only one symptom of how your situation has become appalling. We know that you are being badly treated, that you are neglected and abused. We have invited a social worker, who will come for an inspection tomorrow. We are bringing in also a representative of the city's sanitation services. We want to rid the house of the cats and have it cleaned. During the next month, one member of this group will sleep here in the house every night. We have offered to let Johnny move to the family apartment, which you and Mom have bequeathed to us four in your will. We will do our best to care for Johnny, but this cannot happen at this price! We love you and will do our best to make your life tolerable!

Soon thereafter, most of the cats were removed and a cleaning person was hired. Johnny (at age 66, the oldest "child" in our program) tried to resist, but the social worker involved the police. Ultimately, the family reached a compromise. Johnny was allowed to keep four cats in the house, but weekly visits by the siblings made the father's life conditions much more bearable.

NVR in Psychiatric Contexts

It is common for a family or a therapist to become entangled in questions of diagnosis. Many parents ask us, "What does my child have?" "How do we convince him to take medication?" Often, the adult-child receives psychiatric treatment, but the entrenched dependence remains. The parents are then even more confused. "Should the medication be changed?" or "Can you recommend another psychiatrist?" Wherever possible, we prefer to work with sound clinical data and close psychiatric consultation. However, there are cases where such data or consultation cannot offer a conclusive picture or allow for effective medical treatment, since many adult-children refuse to collaborate with a medical regime or even to meet with a psychiatrist in the first place. Even in such cases, we believe that parents need to learn how to protect themselves and de-accommodate to dysfunctional expectations. The intervention's pace and degree of proposed change might vary according to whether the adult-child suffers from paranoid schizophrenia, OCD or internet addiction, and in absence of such data may be further adjusted to accommodate the greater uncertainty. But in most cases the intervention's core process and goals would remain the same.

By insisting that the adult-child get therapy, the parents rarely get the outcomes they expect. In contrast, in many of our cases, when the parents stopped badgering and accommodating, the adult-child decided to begin treatment. Our program for the parents of children with anxiety disorders who refused therapy had an unexpected result: 70 percent of the children became willing to go to therapy after the parents concluded NVR training (Lebowitz et al., 2014).

Whenever a psychiatrist or other professional caregiver is involved, we try to establish a collaborative relationship. Communicating with the adult-child's psychiatrist, social worker or psychotherapist reduces conflicting messages, diminishing the chaos in the system. Research has shown that increasing "connectedness" (both among professionals and in the family circle) reduces extreme risks such as suicide (Center for Disease Control and Prevention, 2008). Treating families with an adult-child may be highly stressful not only to the parents, but also to the therapist. In our team consultations, we often include psychiatrists and social workers who are familiar with our approach. Sometimes, even when the adult-child refuses to meet with the psychiatrist, a joint consultation may help.

NVR in the Psychiatric Ward

NVR has been shown effective in reducing the use of physical restraint and violence in psychiatric wards (Goddard et al., 2009; van Gink, 2019). NVR in a psychiatric setting can be helpful in other ways too. Hospitalization often occurs when the family can no longer withstand the pressure of the adult-child's problem behaviors. This may happen in the wake of a violent outburst, psychotic outbreak or suicide attempt. Sometimes, it is not the adult-child's condition that worsens, but the family's ability to contain it, for instance because of illness, divorce or financial crisis.

Although the commitment to inpatient psychiatric care is often painful, it may also bring relief, at least in the short run. At first sight, the adult-child's hospitalization opens new horizons, as the mechanisms of accommodation and coercion that prevailed are interrupted by the absence of the adult-child. However, entrenched dependence does not vanish; it simply adapts. Although the bubble that kept parents and adult-child insulated from the outside world bursts at the moment of hospitalization, the process may introduce a new partner, the hospital staff, which may unwittingly feed the dysfunctional dependence.

The relationship between staff and patient is quite different from that between parents and the adult-child. Usually the staff cannot be coerced by the kind of threats or violence to which the parents were subjected, nor does it provide the patient with the services that kept the adult-child protected from unpleasant situations. Although in chronic wards, we sometimes witness a kind of degenerative shelter that reminds us of the chronic environment of some adult-children, this is usually not the case in acute hospital wards where patients do not stay for long. And yet in many cases, hospitalization may be a link in a chain that perpetuates entrenched dependence.

Hospitalization can resemble a thermostat that keeps the family system functioning by keeping it from reaching its breaking point. This can be seen in cases of multiple psychiatric admission (the "revolving door phenomenon"). Many people who are repeatedly hospitalized are adult-children of highly accommodating parents.

Besides serving as a pressure valve for distressed families of adult-children in acute psychiatric conditions, hospitalization may reinforce the dependence bond in other ways. Committing an adult-child to inpatient psychiatric care is often traumatic, both for the parents and the adult-child. Parents often tell us that they would do everything in their power to keep their child from ever having to be institutionalized again. The adult-child, in turn, often blames the parents for the commitment, thus adding a new layer of guilt to the dysfunctional bond.

During the hospital stay, the pressure for accommodation does not stop. The adult-child may flood the parents with telephone calls, complaining about their suffering, mistreatment and horrible life. The parents may receive long and detailed lists of all the things they should bring when they visit. Some parents repeatedly call the hospital in deep worry for their child. Some demand special conditions, accusing the staff of mistreatment and threatening to go to the media or sue the hospital. Staff often react angrily, sometimes blaming the patient for their troubles with the parents. The war of attrition between parents and staff can be deeply damaging. The staff lose influence because they are undermined by the parents, the parents' belief that only they can care for their child is confirmed and the adult-child gains new ways of pressuring the parents into submission.

Conflicts between staff and parents afflict not only psychiatric wards, but also boarding schools and other institutions that cater to the young. We have developed the concept of the *new authority* to adapt to those settings (Omer, 2011). The need for the new concept stems from the fact that traditional authority has become unacceptable, especially in educational and treatment settings. Traditionally, authority was based on distance, strict control and a steep hierarchy. The new authority, in contrast, is based on presence, self-control and support. The concept of the new authority often proves attractive to professionals in institutional settings, because it confers strength in legitimate ways. One of the advantages of the new authority is that it allows for the creation of a common denominator between staff and parents. One message that staff members and parents learn to implement when speaking with each other is that "we are all in the same boat." Here are some illustrations of how the principles of the new authority can be applied when an adult-child is hospitalized.

Presence

The night attendant noticed that a patient in the ward was bullying a new arrival in his room. He told the aggressor that he would keep an eye on him and that the rest of the staff would be notified. In the following hours, he kept coming back to their room, sometimes watching from the door, sometimes sitting on the aggressor's or the victim's bed and asking them calmly if everything was OK. He then reported those occurrences to the morning attendant. The morning attendant told both patients that she had been notified of the incident and said she would stay in contact. Later in the day, the ward director met separately with the aggressor and the victim, telling both that the staff would keep an ear to the ground to guarantee that everything was OK. Through this collective manifestation of presence, the victim felt safer, the aggressor knew he was being observed and the entire staff gained in authority.

Self-Control

The staff of an all-women's ward was trained on how to react when verbally attacked by a very provocative patient. They prepared a note that they kept in their pockets, which said, "I'll discuss this with the other staff members!" Whenever an attendant was verbally attacked by a patient, she would cross her arms and stay silent while looking calmly at the aggressor. If the verbal attack did not subside, she would give the patient the note and walk away. About an hour later, another member of the staff would approach the patient, remind her of what had happened, and tell her, "We've got to find a way for you to stop your outbursts." Before being sent home for the weekend, the patient was called to the director, who reviewed with her the situations in which she had verbally attacked staff members during the week. The director gave her pen and paper and left her alone for 15 minutes to think about ways to change her behavior. When he returned, the patient was sitting in front of a blank sheet. The director said, "We'll continue looking for a solution. Now you can go home." When she returned after the weekend, she no longer berated the staff.

Support

Collaboration with parents (and sometimes with other family members) is one of the important ways in which the new authority in a psychiatric ward differs from the old. The staff says to the parents, "If we join hands, your daughter's stay in the ward will prove helpful both for her and for you." Most parents respond positively, especially as the staff members show that they are interested in resolving the parents' difficulties with their adult-child. Staff meetings with the parents are devoted to formulating ways to protect themselves and reduce accommodation. Plans are devised on how to respond to threats, attacks, repetitive phone calls, endless requests for reassurance and demands for inappropriate services. The parents are invited to participate when the staff implements measures such as sit-ins, documentation and mobilization of support. Parents are offered the staff's support by phone in the weeks following the patient's discharge. In this way, instead of being another link in the chain of dysfunctional dependence, the hospital stay may be a step in the family's emancipation.

In a psychiatric ward, NVR treatment involves all three sides of the "staff–parents–patient" triangle.

Staff and Parents

Some meetings are devoted to the development of a collaborative alliance between the staff and the parents. The staff members who participate in those meetings (usually the patient's doctor, a member of the nursing staff and a social worker) clarify to the parents that they are all partners in the treatment process. The parents are informed and sometimes asked for their opinion about the staff's management of the patient's behavior. Those meetings provide excellent opportunities to prevent conflicts between staff and parents. Parents are often pleasantly surprised to receive emotional and practical support from the staff. The working alliance that emerges from these meetings creates good conditions to continue supporting the parents' further efforts, once the adult-child is back home.

Staff and Patient

Members of the staff meet to discuss dysfunctional dependence patterns between themselves and individual patients. Often the staff is split between those who favor a punitive position and those who favor a protective one. This is reminiscent of the split between the adult-child's parents. The goal of the staff discussion is to develop a group policy of nonescalation and nonaccommodation. Since these skills are relevant for managing the entire ward, they can be learned and discussed during the general staff meetings, thus creating a common language.

Parents and Adult-Child

Meetings between staff and the parents can focus on parental accommodation. Parents are helped to recognize and reduce their accommodating responses both during hospitalization and at home. Weekends at home are important for preparing the parents for their child's discharge. In the weeks following the patient's release, staff remain in touch with the parents by phone, sometimes offering a few booster sessions to help them continue with the de-accommodation that had begun during hospitalization. Sometimes, the staff and the parents agree that the adult-child should not be released home but to another residential facility such as a halfway house or rehabilitative setting.

Lea (34) tried to take her life by jumping from the third story of her parents' home. She underwent multiple surgeries and made an incredible physical recovery. However, a year later she was admitted to a psychiatric ward with depression and suicidal thoughts. Over the next five years, she moved back and forth between the parental home and the hospital ward, gradually accumulating a substantial portfolio of diagnoses and medical treatments. At the time of our intervention, she was described as "suffering from major depression, borderline personality disorder with dependent and narcissistic characteristics and low level of personality organization." She had multiple somatic complaints and functional problems but adamantly refused physiotherapy or rehabilitation. Past treatments included psychiatric medications, Electroconvulsive Therapy and psychotherapy, with no improvement. The staff was used to seeing her come and go. Her communication with her parents and the staff was characterized by endless physical complaints. Instead of talking about her pain, she would whine, groan and sob. Her main grievance was that her pain was not taken seriously. However, when offered a multidisciplinary program for chronic pain, she refused, saying she was too depressed or in too much pain for that.

The life of her parents, Sharon and Tim, was taken up by Lea's needs. For five years, they watched over her continuously, in fear of another suicide attempt, took her to medical appointments, cooked her very special diet and listened to her constant complaints. Sharon gave up her job after Lea called her from work several times, saying that she had swallowed a large quantity of pills. Although it turned out that Lea had lied to get her mother home, Sharon did not feel she could ignore such calls, because it could cost her daughter's life. Sharon and Tim never went out and stopped inviting guests over.

The cycle of hospital commitment and release engendered a dysfunctional dependence pattern among Lea, her parents and the staff. In the hospital, Lea would deliberately call the staff's attention to herself. She would cry loudly, lie on the floor, threaten suicide or accuse the staff of criminal negligence, sometimes writing down her grievances and then reading them aloud. At first, staff members tried to calm her, but with time their responses became blunter. She would then phone her parents, saying she was being mistreated, and demanding to be taken home. The staff avoided the parents, suspecting that they would believe Lea's accusations. The parents would come every day and smuggle in unallowed items. After two or three months of this routine, Lea, her parents and the staff would agree that Lea should be sent home, with bad feelings on all sides. The staff accused the parents of perpetuating Lea's condition and the parents accused the staff of lack of empathy and professionality. Though the parents would swear they would never bring her back, sooner or later the cycle would repeat itself. The chief nurse reflected the generalized despair, saying, "Lea paralyzes everybody with her pain!"

An NVR consultant had been brought to the ward at the initiative of the chief psychiatrist. After the entire staff completed an intensive course in NVR, a plan was devised to cope with Lea's recent rehospitalization. The parents were taken aback when the chief psychiatrist said that they deserved help from the staff, because Lea would not get better unless their own life improved. They were told that Lea's greatest hope for recovery was a good working relationship between them and the staff. The NVR consultant joined the meeting and proposed to the parents a series of sessions with selected staff members, to make sure that any improvements made in the hospital would be maintained after Lea was sent home. After one week, there were already marked improvements in the relationship between parents and staff. In total, there were 21 sessions with the parents: 14 during Lea's hospitalization and 7 after her release.

The first goal was to develop a joint response to Lea's complaints about pain. The parents understood that so long as Lea could get their attention by moaning and whining, she would remain regressed and they would continue to suffer. Lea should be told that both parents and staff knew that her pain was real. However, they could not communicate with her when she "talked pain," that is, when she acted out her pain by crying and groaning. They could only communicate with her if she "talked *about* her pain." The NVR consultant told Lea in the presence of the whole staff that in the future they would be willing to talk to her about her pain, if she were willing to talk in a controlled manner and agreed to look for remedies. However, "talking pain" would no longer be accepted.

The first task of the parents and the staff was to develop their capacity to endure in silence, without admonishing or rushing to help Lea whenever she talked pain. However, when she talked *about* her pain they would start a joint search for possible solutions. If Lea refused to explore treatment options, she should be told, "OK, now you are not ready, so we cannot do anything. Maybe later we can." Three sessions were devoted to help the parents immunize themselves against being consumed by Lea's pain talk. With the staff, they role-played various situations and learned to give Lea messages that expressed their new stance, such as, "In the past I could not stand your crying. Now I know that I can endure it. I know you are in pain and I am ready to talk to you about possible ways of reducing it. But I will no longer continue talking to you when you refuse to consider treatment options." Sometimes the role-playing was so effective that it was exhilarating for the participants. We believe that those moments added emotional depth to the alliance between the parents and the staff.

After a few days, Lea engaged much less in "pain talk," while her readiness to hold normal conversations grew apace. Now, both parents and staff had had a convincing demonstration of the power of a coordinated, consistent and nonescalating strategy.

The reduction in Lea's pain talk and the improvement in communication brought a surprising result: Lea said she wanted to go to a hostel with an intense rehabilitation program instead of coming back home. She said she would never become independent if she continued living with her parents. A few days later, however, Lea changed her mind and asked to be released to her parents' home immediately so that she could prepare for the transfer to the hostel. However, in the staff's opinion, Lea's return home would jeopardize their previous achievements. The parents hesitated. The NVR consultant told the parents that the time had come for a supporters' meeting, since the parents would need support whether they decided to take Lea home or stuck by the decision to keep her in the ward until she was sent to the rehabilitation center.

The meeting included eight supporters (Lea's two brothers and sister-in-law, Sharon's two sisters, their husbands and a close friend of Tim's). The supporters were apprised of the goals and the dilemma over whether Lea should be released home or stay in the ward until she could go directly to the rehabilitation center. All the supporters agreed with the staff. The meeting was a powerful experience for all participants. Lea's younger sister said that this was the first time since Lea's suicide attempt that the parents' needs were taken into consideration. Feeling backed by the supporters, the parents accepted the decision to keep her on the ward. They wrote an announcement, telling Lea that they loved her and would never abandon her, but that they fully agreed with the position of the staff, that she should stay in the hospital until she was transferred to the rehabilitation center.

The parents delivered the announcement with Lea alone, with three members of the staff waiting outside the door. After a few minutes, they came in and found Lea in tears and the parents in deep distress but standing firm. After a while, Lea said, "I see that I have no choice. I must stay here until I go to the rehabilitation center."

The fact that Lea's parents had been able to tell her that she could not come home was a demonstration of their new strength and the effectiveness of their support. In the coming weeks, Lea tried again and again to sway them. Tim and Sharon, however, stood by the decision to keep her in the ward. After four months in the hospital, Lea went to the rehabilitation center. The parents had seven additional sessions to ensure that they would not revert to their pattern of accommodation. Their lives continued to change. They went to the movies and the opera, took a vacation abroad and Sharon trained to become a yoga instructor. They also started visiting and inviting relatives and friends over.

Lea ran away from the rehabilitation center three times. The parents resisted her demands to stay home and convinced her to return to the rehabilitation center. However, it became clear that Lea would leave again. When Lea was finally allowed to come home, she did not stay in bed and did not return to her passive position. There was no more pain talk and the parents did not give up their newfound freedom. Lea took care of her appearance, went out of the house, became willing to use public transportation, had CBT, physiotherapy and hydrotherapy, developed a yearlong intimate relationship, and started meeting with a social worker to get help finding a job. A follow-up five years later showed that the gains had been maintained and there had been no more hospitalization.

7   Survival Mode
The Adult-Child's Experience

Ohad Nahum

This book is about parents of adult-children, their experience, challenges and crucial role in enabling their children's transition from dysfunctional to functional dependence. The therapy presented here is designed to create a safe space for the parents, where their needs would be taken into consideration no less than those of the adult-child. As our work in this parental space progressed, we became more familiar with adult-children. This chapter is devoted to the adult-child's perspective, as we understood it, based on single sessions and other encounters we had with adult-children. As we shall see, these contacts enhanced our work with both the parents and the adult-children.

Previous chapters described how the relational patterns of entrenched dependence evolve and are perpetuated during adolescence and emerging adulthood. The current chapter describes the importance of meeting the adult-child, the conditions that adult-children indicate as contributing factors for their social seclusion, their subjective experience and the internal logic of their passive and withdrawn behavior as a possible means of psychic survival. In addition, this chapter provides some guiding principles for therapeutic work with the adult-child as well as examples of different therapeutic settings in which such therapeutic work takes place.

Meeting the Adult-Child

In our work with adult-children's families, we remained open to three options: inviting the adult-child for a single session; collaborating with the adult-child's existing therapist outside our team; or, when possible, assigning two team members to the case, one to work with the parents and one to work with the adult-child. Adult-children who agreed to come to a single session would be asked whether they would be interested in individual therapy. In case they were, we would usually refer them to a team member other than the one working with their parents. If they were already in therapy, we would ask for permission to contact their therapist. Considering how frequent social withdrawal and therapy refusal are among the population of adult-children whose families come to us, it may not be surprising that most adult-children rejected all three options. In such cases, the parents' therapy proceeded as described in previous chapters. Even in these cases, the insights we gained from meeting other adult-children in a similar predicament were helpful for our work with the parents. Those encounters helped us realize the complex experience of these, often talented, young people, who lived with a continuous sense of entrapment, injury and pain. Parents often mentioned that our description of their child's experience helped them better understand their children emotionally, reconnect with them, overcome communication barriers and reduce escalation cycles. In other words, equipped with both empathic understanding and a course of action, parents felt more anchored.

Developmental Factors of the Adult-Child's Experience

For most adult-children, several early-life conditions that cumulated in and contributed to their current seclusion and social withdrawal can be traced. The most common conditions include developmental vulnerabilities, adverse life experiences and problematic relationships with their parents.

Developmental Vulnerabilities

In our work with adult-children, we often found clear traces of past or ongoing vulnerabilities that undermined the adult-child's sense of competence. For example, ADHD and learning disabilities may lead to scholastic failure and repeated frustration undermining their sense of competence, motivation and self-esteem. Social phobia may precipitate dropout from school or other social institutions. A child with ADHD, learning disabilities or on the autistic spectrum may experience repeated social failures due to a lack of social skills. When these vulnerabilities are met with parental accommodation, a relational pattern of entrenched dependence may develop.

Ronnie (26) had been having extreme emotional outbursts since early childhood. He also had a very low verbal intelligence and severe learning disabilities, making him unable to appropriately express his needs. He responded to frustration by crying and screaming, which would only be relieved when the parents acted to alleviate his stress. Ronnie's father slept with him in his bed, as the family had grown to believe that Ronnie was unable to sleep alone for his anxiety. In adulthood, his outbursts were even more frightening, including suicide threats and gestures, leading to several hospitalizations. His difficulties in discerning what was happening to him probably made the world seem dark and full of terrors, whereas he experienced his parents' total availability to him as the ultimate safe harbor. His screams often sounded like a drowning person's cries for help. Yet, there were situations in which Ronnie could contain his frustration and terror, which opened a window to shades of his experience, other than his flooding anxiety, frustration and terror. For instance, during his school years, his outbursts in school had been rare, and in recent years he would calm down every time he was hospitalized, even before he was medicated. Although flooded with devastating distress at times, it seemed that when Ronnie was with people who did not immediately run to his rescue, he was better able to regulate his emotional state and feel somewhat better. This wider view of Ronnie's inner world (as both capable and anxious) gave his parents some breathing space and hope. They began to realize that if they felt less compelled to rescue Ronnie, he might suffer less anxiety, rather than more.

Adverse Life Experiences

Traumatic experiences, such as death of a family member, being bullied, accidents, illnesses or surgeries may deeply affect the adult-child's inner world. Social traumas such as boycott or bullying were specifically proposed as triggers for the development of *Hikikomori* (Tamaki, 2013). Such experiences may become cumulative, inducing continuous stress that diverts the child from a normative developmental trajectory. We believe that rather than a single traumatic event, it is this gradual buildup of stress in vulnerable children that plays a role in the development of dysfunctional dependence. Examples of adverse events that adult-children mention as milestones on their life trajectory might include family relocation, change of school, romantic rejection, or even a relatively minor biking accident or misfortune. Although these events are no more than what others might consider as unpleasant but normal setbacks, many adult-children experience and describe them as crucial.

Jerry's (21) parents came to therapy one year after he dropped out of college, returned to the parental home and secluded himself in his room. In his single session, he told the therapist that, despite his learning disabilities and limited social skills, he had succeeded in getting through school and holding a part-time job during most of his first two years of college. However, his social isolation, the stress from his studies and his distance from home became more and more difficult to bear. The final straw came with a bitter romantic disappointment at the end of his sophomore year. He fell in love with a girl who seemed to reciprocate his feelings. Unfortunately, when he tried to take it to a romantic level, she rejected him. He tried to take comfort in cannabis, but his situation only deteriorated. Whenever he saw her laughing with friends in the cafeteria, he thought that they were probably laughing at him. This seemed like a replay of his early experiences at school. "I was smart but weird and never belonged," he said at the session. "Kids would tease me constantly, there were always plenty of reasons for them to laugh at me." This experience reinforced his feeling that he was doomed to a life of rejection and social exclusion. For him, shutting himself off was not a choice but a reflection of his lack of choices.

Problematic Relationship with Parents

Relentless criticism, lack of support or parental rejection hinder the development of self-efficacy, damaging the growing child's self-esteem and ability to cope with life's challenges. This is illustrated in Karin's (25) description of her experience with her parents:

My parents were divorced. In my teenage years I would often argue with my mom and she would shout at me things like: "You can take your belongings and get out of our house!" My father wasn't there for me. I would take my stuff and sleep at friends' houses, sometimes for a whole week. OK, I was a rebellious teenager, I did a lot of impulsive and even dangerous things. But my mother tried to control me completely. When I didn't obey, she would kick me out or wouldn't give me money. Even today, when I interview for a part-time job she asks me contemptuously: "Is that a job-interview? Come on, it's a stupid job! Don't you want to do something with yourself?"

Karin's mother did not take issue with Karin's description. She felt deeply guilty about her hurtful remarks. She described the continuous worry in which they lived, as Karin associated with bad people, came home drunk, and stole her money again and again. The event in which the mother had ordered Karin to leave the house happened only once, after Karin had reacted to the mother's attempts to set boundaries by physically attacking her and throwing the mother's cell phone into the toilet.

In such cases, it is not the therapists' role to sort out what happened. However, if the child's and the parents' therapists collaborate, they can validate the subjective experience of both sides in ways that may open new possibilities. In this case the parents' therapist said to the mother:

I can see that you feel guilty about the way you sometimes responded to Karin. Even now, you may respond problematically when she has good news, like trying to get a job. In fact, both Karin and you have short fuses. Our goal is to help you feel less helpless, more supported and able to act constructively. In our joint work you will learn not to give in to Karin's provocations nor pander to her negative inclinations. On the contrary, we will find ways in which you can resist her while supporting her. Parents who stop being helpless may also become able to admit past mistakes. They then do it out of a position of strength and not of weakness. This could be an important experience for you and your daughter.

Karin's therapist said to Karin:

I have no doubt that you felt brutally criticized and rejected by your mother. I know from her therapist's reports how helpless she often felt, especially in your adolescence. I also know she now acknowledges her past mistakes, and I know how guilty she feels about her negative reactions towards you. Your mother wants to be able to create a less explosive relationship between you two. She loves you and cares for you and wants to make things different from her side. Would you be willing to give her a chance?

Such reframes are often the result of the collaboration between the adult-child's and the parents' therapists. They indicate how empathy can be reintroduced into the family system. Regret for past actions can then be expressed without the need for inappropriate compensation. Such reparation which decreases the adult-child's sense of estrangement toward their family may help to establish a less alienated stance toward the world.

The Adult-Child Experience

The Adult-Child's Sense of Incompetence

The adverse relations and life experiences described in the previous section, combined with structural vulnerabilities, can lead adult-children to gradually lose their sense of competence or self-efficacy. Adult-children often tell us how they lost faith in their ability to steer their life course and how incapable they felt of rising to the challenges that awaited them outside the parental home. Little by little even simple routines became ordeals. This experience of incompetence can gradually crystallize into learned helplessness, passivity and despair, accompanied by self-contempt. These feelings fuel the tendency to avoid any challenging situation since even the most mundane tasks seem not only impossible but highly risky to the self – a painful confirmation of one's incompetence. Tasks such as coping with bureaucracy or undertaking professional training become well-nigh impossible.

The adult-child appears to be unmotivated. However, adult-children are powerfully motivated by the need to avoid further failures and painful rejections as a way of self-preservation. Maintaining their self-withdrawal is therefore the only option they believe to be possible. Even when they seem resourceful, their resources are often invested in preserving things as they are. This is frequently accompanied by a defensive attitude, such as blaming their parents for their difficulties. Some even blame their parents for their poor genetic endowment or for having brought them into this world.

Even the shadow of success may become a threat to their hard-won equilibrium. That is why, when they are offered a job interview, a new study program or a social opportunity, they often use expressions like "I'm a lost cause!" "It's too late!" or "Who will want someone like me?" These reactions are weapons to fend off opportunities that they see as existential hazards and deep threats to their sense of self.

It is noted that in apparent contrast to their social and practical ineptitude, many adult-children develop impressive knowledge and proficiency in some areas. They can be experts on politics, jazz or astrophysics, or develop considerable knowledge in origami, the history of philosophy or advanced computer gaming. Their skills provide them with a sense of self-worth and protection. Unfortunately, they often keep those aptitudes hermetically sealed from any application in the real world.

Shame

Constant shame may be the most pivotal feeling in the adult-child's emotional world. Anxiety, depression, anger and spite all play their roles at different times, but probably nothing is as all-pervasive as shame. Hanging on to self-withdrawal may provide some sense of safety, but at the cost of a deep sense of shame.

John (27) had never worked. After spending more than six years studying toward an undergraduate degree, and failing the same single course multiple times, he gave up and retired to his parents' home, where he spent most of his time playing computer games. He seldom left the house and cut off all contact with friends, sharing with the therapist his sense that he could not see them anymore because they would inquire about his life. He avoided meeting with relatives, so as not to be asked about work or studies. "I'm ashamed. Everybody else is out of my league."

Shame is a deeply painful experience, which is often accompanied by a desire to vanish (as reflected in everyday language "I am so ashamed I wanted to bury myself!"). This wish to hide and vanish is central to the lives of many adult-children. That is why so many of them prefer to stay up at night and sleep during the daytime. As one of the adult-children we interviewed described it, "I'm ashamed to invite friends, I am ashamed to meet with my family, I have no answers, they all did things with their lives and I didn't." The wish to hide may intensify into a motivation for self-erasure, sometimes leading to suicidal ideation. Shame may grow into self-hatred, as illustrated in the following quotes from two adult-children we interviewed:

Sue (29): "I hate myself; I don't understand how all this time went by and I did nothing! It's not only that I haven't achieved anything, there is simply no chance that I ever will ... "
   Allan (20): "I don't deserve anything, I'm a total failure, I am nothing, I am zero."

For many adult-children, this kind of self-talk would be unbearable. One of the ways in which they protect themselves is by adopting a high social conscience. This allows them to feel some sense of worth by devaluating the people around them, thus reducing their own sense of inferiority.

Jonathan (36), who did not work or study, devoted most of his days to managing an internet forum on rescuing abandoned dogs. He would go out only at night looking for strays, avoiding any interaction with former friends or family members. When he talked about others, particularly his parents, he would express righteous anger at their alleged cruelty and indifference. In those moments he felt pride at having turned his back on a world which he morally despised.

One might be surprised by the discrepancy between Jonathan's concern for abandoned dogs and his cruel accusations against his parents. This discrepancy reflects his identification with the weak and oppressed. Often, these high moral aspirations may indicate the difficulty these young adults experience in achieving the compromises that might allow them to participate in the actual adult world. The gap between their ideals and the outside world may widen to the point of becoming an unbridgeable chasm. In this process, the entrance point to the actual world recedes into the distance.

This paralysis is reminiscent of the existential trap depicted in Kafka's short story, *Before the law.* In the story, a man from the country seeks to pass through a gate that bars the entrance to "the law." In our interpretation, "the law" is the state of things as they should be, so entering "the law" would be tantamount to fulfilling one's destiny and realizing one's potential and high ideals. The gate is kept by a guard, and the man from the country waits for the guard to allow him passage. This never happens, but the man keeps waiting. He spends his best years waiting. The guard explains that he is only the least of the guards, implying a never-ending chain of guards to beat, with each guard more powerful and frightening than the last. The man imagines the endless obstacles that stand in his way. Any significant action is seen as requiring Herculean strength, with every new step being more difficult than the last. As one of our clients described it: "I don't want to try and suffer just to find out that the next step will require even more effort, and the next one, even more so." In Kafka's story, when the man from the country is about to die after years of waiting, the guard bends over him and, so as to reach him through his failing hearing, shouts to him that the gate that he had not passed through was intended only for him and now, when he dies, the gate will be closed. His last vision is of the bright light that shines behind the slowly closing doors.

Most adult-children, however, do not wait in quiet resignation but are in constant inner turmoil. Even when they seem placid and content, they are consumed with shame. To ward off their experience of shame, they may sink into substance abuse or addiction to computer games. However, they must be left alone to achieve this relief, for every contact with others renews their shame. Indeed, many of them protest to their parents, "I don't want anything from you! Just leave me alone!" At times, some of them have recourse to another palliative: attacking and shaming the other.

Uri (42) would often accuse his father, who had retired from public office a year before, "You are a parasite! You and those like you are the cause of our economic crisis! Because of people like you, there is no chance that others may earn a decent living through normal jobs. Now you want me to work so that the country may pay for your pension! But I'm not going to work minimum wage just to support your parasitic lifestyle!" The fallacious nature of this argument did not prevent Uri from reiterating it.

In Uri's case, diverting his attacks on the self toward his father provided temporary relief and refuge from his inner shame and painful affects.

In other cases, the attacks on the surroundings are hidden and implicit, taking place mostly in the mind of the adult-child and directed not concretely at the parents, but at values such as injustice, capitalism, materialism or social indifference. Though many of these claims may be valid, adult-children use them as an agenda that explains their distaste toward the world and justifies their self-withdrawal. This deepens the gap between the inside and the outside, between the adult-child and others, and between the illusory control in escaping into their room and the total lack of control they experience in the outside world.

Alienation toward the environment also functions as a defense against social rejection. Moving away from those who reject us is a universal mechanism of self-protection. When feeling inadequate, rejected and cast out, many adult-children regain control by rejecting those who have rejected or even *might* reject them.

Ariel (27) has withdrawn into his home since finishing his military service – where he had held a deeply frustrating job for which he felt overqualified. His attempts to change his placement fell on deaf ears and his commanders worsened his troubles by threatening to "straighten him up." Ariel saw his army experience as a defining moment. He would no longer be a pawn of the society that had oppressed and humiliated him. He said, "Society forces people to serve in the army and, if you don't fit into their framework, then you're stuck, and no one cares. Society will continue to crush us all if we allow what happened to me to go on happening. Therefore, I simply refuse to work, to contribute, to be a part of the system."

Similar experiences and justifications of self-withdrawal have been documented by observers of the *Hikikomori* phenomenon described in Japan and other countries (Tajan, 2015).

So far, we have discussed how adult-children's early vulnerabilities, stressful life-events and negative interactions induce a sense of incompetence and a chronic sense of failure. New opportunities foreshadow additional disappointments and are hence experienced as threats. To protect themself, the adult-child retreats into passivity, often blaming others for their plight as a maneuver to escape the tormenting inner shame. This shame may explain the ferocious attacks of some of those adult-children against their parents. The serious gap between their passivity in the world and the fury they display at home gives us a hint of their need to compensate for their sense of helplessness and inferiority.

Survival Mode

We have seen how the interaction between objective vulnerabilities and difficulties, adverse life-events and negative relations with significant others may lead to a feeling of incompetence and deep shame, and to self-withdrawal as an act of self-preservation. Any initiative in the real world is out of the question, signifying only further rejection and criticism. If self-esteem is the fuel that allows us to propel ourselves through the world, from the adult-child's point of view there are only a few drops left at their disposal. The adult-child is operating under a conservative "survival mode" – any action outside their shelter is like trying to cross the desert in a car with the fuel warning light on. Keeping their rule in the little realm of their room, maintaining their protected conditions and the parental services they receive, and sometimes manifesting their precarious sense of special value against their parents or society at large represent the act of psychological survival. Ineffective as this may be, extreme passivity, self-seclusion and imperviousness to all demands and expectations represent an attempt to regain a minimal sense of competence. Even more tragically, some of these young adults become defensively invested in their own incompetence. Proving they are hopeless might become their triumph, by which they defeat even the most diligent would-be rehabilitators. Their Pyrrhic victory, however, is but a gloss for their overwhelming and painful sense of shame.

The Therapeutic Encounter with the Adult-Child

Considering how pervasive shame is in the experience of adult-children and how deeply it can hurt their eventual social reintegration, it seems that reducing shame should be a high priority in their therapy. However, adult-children usually feel they have a lot to be ashamed of. An attitude of therapeutic acceptance and unconditional positive feedback may simply not suffice, so long as the adult-child continues living in passivity and dependence. One possible way of addressing the problem is our distinction between "destructive" and "constructive" shame. Destructive shame leads to disconnection; constructive shame creates options for reconnection. When shame is experienced in a context of exclusion or humiliation it is profoundly damaging. In contrast, shame that is experienced in a context of support can be a bridge to renewed belonging. The central question for therapy is: How can the experience of shame be *transformed* so that it becomes constructive and connecting rather than destructive and disconnecting?

Transforming Shame through a New Narrative

After his parents came to consultation with another NVR therapist from our team, Alex (30) agreed to come to see me and remained in individual therapy for nine months. Over the past seven years, Alex had studied toward a degree in a demanding profession but avoided taking the final exams. This experience left him with an overwhelming sense of defeat. He described himself as being always slow at school and easily hurt in his relationships with others. He described his parents as critical and disparaging. They often tried to motivate him but in ways he experienced as belittling. Gradually, his feelings of incompetence and fear of being hurt, combined with his sensitive character, led him to a preference for a risk-free and limited life of seclusion. "I have to avoid situations in which I feel something," he said, "because feelings are always negative. I'd like to press 'delete' over all the feelings I have."

He described his shame when a childhood friend found him on Facebook and invited him to his wedding. "I don't know what to answer him," Alex said. "I don't want to go out and deal with any questions, I haven't met him and my friends in five years. No . . . I don't think I can go . . . what can I tell them?" Later in the therapy, he said, "How is it possible to get close to anyone? How will I explain that I have done nothing all these years?"

The therapist replied:

"I understand your shame and your sense of failure. And yet, in today's world, many young people spend a lot of time in all kinds of strange pursuits before choosing a vocation and define their life path. Many spend years 'just searching for themselves.' Perhaps we can think together about how you got lost in the labyrinth of your search. And then maybe we'll know what you can tell somebody else about your 'lost years'?"

Instead of immediately trying to alleviate Alex's sense of shame, the therapist validated his feelings but proposed an alternative life-narrative, in which Alex might have gotten lost searching for himself like many emerging adults. Creating a new narrative for Alex's "lost years" could be an important therapeutic goal. In subsequent sessions, Alex and the therapist worked together to build this narrative, which, without distorting or idealizing his situation, was richer and more multifaceted than his self-description as a total loser.

Alex had become stuck in his academic studies. His stubborn pursuit of a goal that was probably unsuited for him might have been a tragic mistake, but his determination showed he had a fighting side to him. The therapist and Alex talked about young people who suddenly found out that they had been on the wrong path for years, others who went for endless trips around the world or those who sought salvation in drugs or cults.

Gradually a new life-narrative emerged, as Alex began referring to himself with compassion saying, "I'm different and slow, I've always taken a long time to decide and adapt. It's a pity that it took me so long, but I've suffered enough. It's time to try something else. Now I'll go slow and be more careful. I won't throw myself headlong in a direction that is wrong for me." This new formulation set the stage for an attitude of careful experimentation that was a good antidote for his withdrawal.

Transforming Shame and Reducing Anxiety by Gradual Exposure

Renarrating one's life, however, may not be enough to change the adult-child's life course. Anxiety and shame keep the adult-child in avoidance. New experiences are needed to gradually reduce anxiety and avoidance, transforming the sense of shame into a sense of struggle.

For an adult-child who is steeped in avoidance, every action may look like a climb up Mount Everest. Therefore, even small steps in the right direction may trigger a process of change, which in turn feeds the new life-narrative that is gradually being developed. This process is known as gradual exposure in

CBT, taking small steps to restore a sense of competence. For an adult-child who has not left their room for months, even walking around the family home or condo at night or spending 30 minutes on a park bench with a cell phone may be a beginning. These tiny steps have a paradoxical effect, a strategy we call "the homeopathic principle."

The paradoxical effect of the homeopathic principle manifests itself in that some of these initial exposure tasks, which elicit shame in the adult-child, are curative in small and controlled doses. This may give a good opportunity for the therapist to develop a discussion about aspirations. This was the case with Alex, who had to adapt the aspirations that had led him to try again and again to complete a course of studies to which he was ill-suited.

In discussing the significance of small exposure tasks, the therapist emphasized that even a small achievement is worth infinitely more than none. The therapist may say to the adult-child: "It takes double courage to do this: The courage to undertake any task at all, and the courage to undertake such a *small* task." Accepting to perform a very small task is an important event in the transformation of shame. Accepting a very modest step as a significant achievement represents the willingness to begin acting despite feelings of shame.

The gradual return to an active routine triggered a change in Alex's aspirations. He learned to settle for more realistic goals without feeling humiliated. Even though the exposure was very gradual, the tasks became more and more meaningful. He began going out for a walk twice a week, reconnected with some old friends by email and, after a few months, began searching for a job. Each small step helped transform his life-narrative in ways he could eventually share with family and friends. Alex began telling his family that he was learning from past mistakes and had been wrong to insist on an inappropriate course of study for so long. After 8 months he was working part-time. This allowed him to move into a small studio flat. After a discussion between Alex's therapist and the parents' therapist, the parents agreed to cover Alex's rent for three years, but he had to pay his bills. Though shaky at first, this arrangement lasted.

At the end of therapy, Alex said that the most difficult part had been to reintroduce himself into the world. He said that what had helped him most was the understanding that many young people find it exceedingly difficult to find their path. The idea of slowness had also been hugely important for him. He said that these insights had helped him bear his shame and to move on at his own pace.

Transforming Shame by Reconnection

There is a marked difference between shame that is experienced in the context of social withdrawal and shame that is lived in the process of social reconnection. The transition between the two is possibly the deepest transformation many adult-children undergo on their way to recovery. For this reason, helping the adult-child move out of isolation is the highest of therapeutic priorities.

An adult-child who is willing to come to therapy is usually more amenable to such an endeavor than one who refuses any therapeutic help. In cases of complete refusal, the young person's hope of emerging from isolation depends almost exclusively upon the parents' readiness to involve a support group. In contrast, an adult-child who comes to therapy has already taken the first step in establishing contact, even if only in the highly protected context of psycho-therapy. The therapist may stress this point, saying for instance,

Your *willingness* to talk to me about your difficulties cannot be taken for granted. Many young people in your situation don't dare to make this step. But probably the best chance for a change is if you could use our meetings as support and I could serve as a bridge to help you negotiate the abyss that keeps you away from people.

The transformation of shame that occurs when the adult-child starts meeting with others is achieved, among other reasons, by exploring these experiences in therapy. We have already seen how the creation of a new life-narrative helped Alex communicate differently with his parents and others. Each of these contacts was grist for the therapeutic mill, allowing for a productive discussion about the changing nature of Alex's shame. The very distinction between "constructive" and "destructive" shame became a significant personal resource in Alex's coping repertoire.

Reconnection should be gradual, like any other process of exposure. A young person who is entrenched in social avoidance must feel supported in taking the first steps in this direction. The therapist may inquire whether the adult-child has any contacts, even anonymous, for instance through the Internet. The possibility of joining a therapy group for social phobia, or an internet forum of lonely young people, people who have long been out of work or young people addicted to gaming can be discussed.

Some of the most significant contacts are those in which relationships that were important in the past but long-neglected are tentatively reinstated. The therapist may play a bridging role in planning for possible ways of establishing contact and role-playing scripts for eventual meetings.

Meeting the Adult-Child in the Context of an Ongoing Parent Therapy

Adult-children who are willing to either come to a single session with the parents' therapist or undertake therapy for themselves may open options for change that are not available for those who refuse all contact. However, even those who reject a meeting with a therapist may not be completely insulated from attempts to reach out to them. Thus, many adult-children, who had previously been impervious to any offer of help, responded well when positively addressed by a supporter. Moreover, as the parents gradually reduced their accommodation, some adult-children who had previously refused therapy changed their minds. Some may demand as a quid pro quo that the parents stop their acts of resistance. We warn parents that agreeing to such a demand might severely damage both the prospects of the child's therapy and their parent therapy. Some adult-children, however, decide to go to therapy, even though the parents refuse to stop the process of de-accommodation. Studies using the NVR approach (Lebowitz et al., 2014) found that most children who had refused professional help in the past became willing to undergo therapy once the parents stopped accommodating them. This holds also for adult-children, though the proportion is probably smaller.

Even a single session with the parents' therapist can be of help in some ways. It may allow for a fuller picture of the adult-child's condition and family constellation; the adult-child may get a better understanding both of the parents' endeavor, as well as their care and worry; and new channels for help and mediation may be opened.

Although the parents describe their child's situation at length, there is nothing better than a direct encounter to provide the parents' therapist with a good picture of the adult-child, their internal state and their interpersonal relations. Family dynamics are often characterized as a dance. So now, instead of imagining the role and steps of the child in the family dance, the therapist gets to meet the dancer. The parents are also reassured when the therapist can form a first-hand impression of the adult-child, and their strengths, vulnerabilities and capabilities. The session also allows an empathic and a richer perspective on the adult-child's clinical condition. Although the session does not proceed along the lines of a diagnostic interview, the fact that the therapist can observe the adult-child may lead to a tentative diagnosis. In some of our cases, this has opened new options for treatment. Finally, the therapist may be able to explain the parents' intentions to the adult-child.

Adult-children usually react positively to the declared goal of reducing escalation. Sometimes, they even adopt this goal for themselves. The therapist makes it clear to the adult-child that the parents' therapy does not aim at controlling the adult-child, but at helping the parents develop self-control and provide appropriate support. An additional potential gain of the meeting with the adult-child has to do with the involvement of supporters. If the atmosphere of the meeting is positive, the therapist can tell the adult-child that they might also profit from the involvement of selected supporters. For instance, they might profit from their ability to mediate between them and their parents. This presentation of the supporter group may reduce the tendency of the adult-child to view the supporters as representatives of the society who do not give up on them, rather than viewing them as totally hostile to their interests.

A Single Meeting with the Adult-Child

Ezra (36) lived with his father, who completely supported him financially, although he worried that he could not afford to continue doing so indefinitely. His mother had died in a car accident several years earlier, an event that intensified Ezra's seclusion. According to Ezra's father, his wife had been the only person who "was able to sometimes drag him out or make him do something." He told the therapist his son suffered from deep anxiety and compulsive hoarding and seemed increasingly preoccupied and anxious during the day. Ezra's family doctor prescribed him Clonex for when the anxiety intensified to the point of panic attacks. Although lately his anxiety had soared, Ezra refused to see a psychiatrist.

Initially, since Ezra refused any treatment, his father arrived for consultation. After a few sessions, he began to resist Ezra's compulsive patterns that took place outside his room in the shared home space, while at the same time making sure to offer positive gestures and support. He delivered Ezra the following empathic message:

Son, in recent years you have suffered from fears and compulsions that have restricted your life and mine to an impossible degree. Initially, I thought that if I gave you time things would get better, but the situation got worse. Mom's loss was a terrible blow for both of us, but now I've decided I don't want to lose you too! I can see that your suffering increased lately, I am worried, and I started attending counseling sessions in the hope of changing the situation at home. I'm afraid I don't understand everything you are going through. I would be happy if you joined me for a session with the therapist I'm meeting so he might help me understand what is going on and how I can provide appropriate assistance.

Ezra agreed and arrived together with his father. Five minutes into the session, he requested to speak to the therapist in private. In the conversation, it soon became clear that Ezra was in terrible pain, suffering not only from deep anxiety but also from a paranoid condition that included fear of being attacked on the street. He therefore carried a knife with him everywhere, including to the meeting with the therapist. After Ezra briefly described his feelings, the therapist told him:

Ezra, I realize that you are suffering – you are haunted by horrible fears, to the point of feeling in constant and extreme danger. You do not deserve to suffer like this, you deserve to feel good and take care of yourself. But I also understand that you don't have the strength to do it by yourself right now, and you need help. Your condition is not only impossible for you but also for your father. He is concerned about you and wants to find you the best treatment. I think that your suffering has intensified to the point that justifies spending some time in psychiatric daycare, so that a better therapy may be found for you – a better treatment than the Clonex, which isn't delivering the relief you need. Would you be willing to visit the psychiatric daycare center together with your father and try, only try, what they might offer? I understand that this option may provoke anxiety, but at least your suffering will have now meaning and purpose – to reduce the burden of your anxiety and feel safe in the world again.

After the therapist promised to speak to the psychiatrist, Ezra agreed to give it a try. This was the first time Ezra had agreed to see a psychiatrist. The psychiatrist offered him hospitalization for a few days until the antipsychotics took effect. Ezra agreed. After a short hospitalization, his paranoia and anxiety subsided. In the meantime, the father took steps to de-accommodate to Ezra's compulsions and hoardings. Ezra's functioning gradually improved. His hospitalization made him eligible for a disability pension from Social Security and for several protected jobs, which he explored with the social worker at the psychiatric daycare center.

Although not all single meetings with adult-children end up in such collaboration and willingness to get therapeutic help, Ezra's case illustrates the importance of reaching out to the adult-child, as even a single meeting can serve as a turning point when conducted with hope and empathy.

Parallel Therapy with the Parents and the Adult-Child

Hal (35) was the youngest of three siblings and the only one still living with his parents. He was a quiet, agreeable, introverted guy with a relaxed pace and temperament, at least to the outside observer. Hal avoided social interactions and, apart from his parents, he did not keep any social contacts. He worked at part-time jobs, which did not allow him to live on his own and did not promote any social interactions. He had been studying toward Certification as a Public Accountant (CPA) but had failed the certification exams three times. Hal intended to continue living with his parents, even though they felt that his stay at home was detrimental to his functioning, sense of self-worth and his chances of independent life.

Hal's parents went through the early phases in our therapy and succeeded in involving supporters and reducing some of their inappropriate services. Gradually, they concluded that it was time for Hal to move out and that they would help him financially. They set a date for his move, stressing that they would still be there to help him. One of the supporters proposed to Hal that he get therapy from someone who specialized in cases like his. Hal agreed to go to therapy and consented that his therapist exchange information with his parents' therapist. This opened the way for a fruitful collaboration between them.

Among other reasons, Hal hoped that by coming to therapy he would show his parents his goodwill and perhaps get them to reconsider asking him to leave their home. Despite this ulterior motive, his engagement in therapy was positive. Hal's therapist was impressed with his sensitivity and generosity. Surprisingly, he drew courage from his parents' encouragement to move forward but was constantly afraid of disappointing them. He was ashamed of having failed his certification exams and ruminated harshly about his missed opportunities. Despite that, he succeeded in undertaking some steps he had previously avoided.

He and his therapist discussed the way he had approached his exams in the past and made a detailed plan to prepare for them in a better way. He agreed to prepare in advance for job interviews. The two made a point of developing scripts in which his application was refused. After a couple of months, Hal found a better job.

However, when the deadline that the parents had set for his leaving home approached, Hal felt he was still unable to sustain himself, even with his parents' help. He said he understood his parents but that the pace was wrong. In his therapist's talks with the parents' therapist, the groundwork was laid for renegotiating the process of leaving home. Hal explained to his parents that he would continue working but that preparing for an additional attempt to pass his exam was also stressful. The parents agreed to postpone his moving out.

Hal left his parents' home for a small apartment six months after the original date that the parents had set. A year later he passed the exam and began working as an accountant. Hal's therapy continued for two additional years. In Hal's case, the collaboration between the two therapists had allowed for the development of an appropriate pace that proved acceptable to Hal and his parents.

These different venues (single meeting, parallel therapy within our team and collaboration with the adult-child's therapist) for getting to know the adult-children whose parents were undergoing NVR treatment in our team have greatly enriched our intervention. Besides, some of these ventures have proved very helpful for a minority of adult-children to begin their journey of self-liberation from their tormenting avoidance, withdrawal and seclusion. More resources should be invested in motivating adult-children to consider therapy. We believe that our intervention is one factor that can help lower treatment refusal rates.

Conclusion

This book introduced the notion of AED as a family systemic condition linked to a failure to emerge into adulthood. It also introduced our treatment approach for helping the parents of adult-children. To our knowledge, this is the first work proposing a systematic treatment for a condition that is probably spreading worldwide. As a pioneering work, it must leave behind it a long trail of unanswered questions for further exploration. We sincerely hope that the following points will inspire clinicians and researchers to investigate this as yet uncharted field.

- *Entrenched Dependence and NEET:* Almost all the adult-children we saw over 10 years of work could be considered "inactive NEET," that is, were not in employment, education or training, nor actively searching for any. According to OECD estimates, in the OECD zone alone, there are about 28 million inactive NEET (OECD, 2016). What part of this population can be considered adult-children in our sense? What is the relationship between entrenched dependence and the NEET demographic?

- *Predisposing Factors of Entrenched Dependence:* What factors predispose individuals and families to become governed by dependence–accommodation relationship patterns? Learning more about these factors might eventually help assess a given young person's risk of emergence failure.

- *Prevention of Emergence Failure:* In Chapter 7, we pointed out several risk factors in childhood and adolescence that are probably linked to the development of Adult Entrenched Dependence. Research into these conditions could help assess the risk of emergence and failure, thus helping develop preventive interventions.

- *AED and Psychopathology:* As we noted in Chapter 1, the interactional patterns of AED are highly similar across a wide range of diagnoses. In our experience, once the dependence–accommodation cycle was interrupted, the adult-child and the family atmosphere improved markedly, no matter the diagnosis. Thus, AED seems to be a trans-diagnostic condition (Shimshoni et al., 2019). Despite this, a question remains on the extent and ways in which different diagnoses impose unique constraints or parameters on the development, configuration and treatment of entrenched dependence.

- *The Efficacy of NVR Therapy for AED:* Various modes are used for the delivery of NVR for AED. One variation involves only the parents. In another variety, both parents and adult-children are clients (treated by different therapists). An important question for research regards the efficacy of treatment when the adult-child is an active client or only a passive receiver.
- *AED and the Public Interest:* It would be mistaken to assume that AED is enabled purely by intrafamilial factors. Many macro-social, economic, cultural and normative influences are also at play. Examples include sociocultural discourses of privacy, independence, self-realization, self-regulation and liberalism; the demographics and culture of emerging adulthood; economic recession, unemployment and high entry barriers into the job market; and the lack of public awareness regarding AED. Research should help clarify what can be done on a social level to help families of adult-children to identify their problem and find ways of minimizing it.

We would like to conclude with some reflections on our 20 years of experience in helping parents of difficult children through NVR.

Parents who are coached in NVR must find courage to do many things they never dared to do. This is true about the parents of children in all age groups, but much more so about the parents of adult-children. Therapists, too, need courage to guide a process that is often fraught with strong emotions, dire threats and potentially hurtful acts. The task would seem totally daunting, were it not for what we know about NVR both in the sociopolitical and the family contexts.

Non-Violent Resistance did not evolve to serve the brave, but those who had hitherto bowed to their fate as if it were part of the natural order. In the sociopolitical arena, NVR is typically launched by an initial act of refusal, which welds together the community of resistors. The resistors' courage surprises even themselves. The same is true about the family context. Parents are amazed to discover that they can act. Therapists who are new to NVR are also often stunned by the parents' courage and by their own guiding role. Having experienced the inspiring effects of a supporters' gathering, a sit-in with a violent child or a telephone round with an adolescent at risk (Omer, 2004b; in press), therapists learn to believe in the parents' capacity to make a stand against the flood of dangers that threaten to overwhelm the child and the family. This courage proves contagious. Eventually, the child "catches courage" too, becoming better able to cope with their own life challenges.

The condition of AED represents a total breakdown of courage in the family. It also challenges some of traditional psychotherapy's most cherished values. Very often, chronic violence, abuse and stagnation in such families go hand in hand with total secrecy. However, traditional psychotherapy as we know it upholds privacy as an absolute value, which may be just the opposite of what these families need. In addition, parents of adult-children are firmly bound to their subservient role by their narrative of total responsibility. Yet this narrative is quite compatible and often abetted by current therapeutic discourses of parenthood, which reinforce the belief in the total responsibility, if not downright guilt, of the parents. Finally, many parents of adult-children see the lack of dialogue between them and their children as the chief problem, entertaining hopes of achieving this dialogue through therapy. Although therapy can and should aim for dialogue, an absolute trust in its all-healing power may be detrimental, especially when continuing the conversation postpones or blocks the path for action. We believe that the tools and values of NVR may help prevent these pitfalls. We are very encouraged by the reactions of parents to our program, as despair becomes suffused with hope and paralysis turns into action. The moment of deepest transformation is witnessed at the supporters' gathering. When the weak "I" of the parent becomes the strong "We" of a caring and committed group, everything changes. We believe that these small communities are the crucible where fear is welded into courage.

Bibliography

Adrian, M. (2018). The collaborative assessment and management of suicidality: Application and adaptations with youth. *Journal of the American Academy of Child and Adolescent Psychiatry, 57* (Suppl 10). https://doi.org/10.1186/s12888-020-02589-x

Alon, N., & Omer, H. (2006). *The psychology of demonization: Promoting acceptance and reducing conflict.* Lawrence Erlbaum Associates Publishers.

Angone, P. (2014). What is emerging adulthood? And why it explains millennials in their 20s. Internet blog. https://allgroanup.com/featured/what-is-emerging-adulthood-and-why-it-explains-your-twenties/

Arnett, J. J. (2000). Emerging adulthood. A theory of development from the late teens through the twenties. *The American Psychologist, 55*(5), 469–480. https://doi.org/10.1037/0003-066X.55.5.469 PMID:10842426

Arnett, J. J. (2004). *Emerging adulthood: The winding road from the late teens through the twenties.* Oxford University Press.

Arnett, J. J., & Schwab, J. (2012). *The Clark University Poll of Emerging Adults: Thriving, struggling, and hopeful.* Clark University.

Arnett, J. J., & Schwab, J. (2014). *Becoming established adults: Busy, joyful, stressed – and still dreaming big. The Clark University Poll of Established Adults Ages 25–39.* Clark University.

Bateson, G. (1972). *Steps to an ecology of mind.* Ballantine Books.

Ben-Porath, D. (2010). Dialectical Behavior Therapy applied to parent skills training: Adjunctive treatment for parents with difficulties in affect regulation. *Cognitive and Behavioral Practice, 17*, 458–465. https://doi.org/10.1016/j.cbpra.2009.07.005

Carli, V., Hoven, C. W., Wasserman, C. et al. (2014). A newly identified group of adolescents at "invisible" risk for psychopathology and suicidal behavior: Findings from the SEYLE study. *World Psychiatry, 13*: 78–86. doi:10.1002/wps.20088

Carlton, P., & Deane, F. P. (2000). Impact of attitudes and suicidal ideation on adolescents' intentions to seek professional psychological help. *Journal of Adolescence, 23*(1), 35–45. doi:10.1006/jado.1999.0299

Center for Disease Control and Prevention [CDC] (2008). Strategic direction for the prevention of suicidal behavior: Promoting individual, family, and community connectedness to prevent suicidal behavior. Report. www.sprc.org/resources-programs/strategic-direction-prevention-suicidal-behavior-promoting-individual-family-and

Daniel, S. S., & Goldston, D. B. (2009). Interventions for suicidal youth: A review of the literature and developmental considerations. *Suicide & Life-Threatening Behavior, 39* (3), 252–268. www.ncbi.nlm.nih.gov/pmc/articles/PMC2819305/ PMID:19606918

Diamond, G. M., Diamond, G. S., Levy, S., Closs, C., Ladipo, T., & Siqueland, L. (2012). Attachment-based family therapy for suicidal lesbian, gay, and bisexual adolescents: A treatment development study and open trial with preliminary findings. *Psychotherapy*, *49*(1), 62–71. https://doi.org/10.1037/a0026247 PMID:22181026

Diamond, G. S., Wintersteen, M. B., Brown, G. K. et al. (2010). Attachment-based family therapy for adolescents with suicidal ideation: A randomized controlled trial. *Journal of the American Academy of Child and Adolescent Psychiatry*, *49*, 122–131. PMID:20215934

Dube, S. R., Anda, R. F., Felitti, V. J. et al. (2001). Childhood abuse, household dysfunction, and the risk of attempted suicide throughout the life span: Findings from the Adverse Childhood Experiences Study. *Journal of the American Medical Association*, *286*(24), 3089–3096. https://doi.org/10.1001/jama.286.24.3089 PMID:11754674

Fergusson, D. M., Woodward, L. J., & Horwood, L. J. (2000). Risk factors and life processes associated with the onset of suicidal behaviour during adolescence and early adulthood. *Psychological Medicine*, *30*(1), 23–39. https://doi.org/10.1017/S00 3329179900135X PMID:10722173

Franc, N., & Omer, H. (2017). *Accompagner les parents d'enfants tyranniques*. Dunod. www.dunod.com/sciences-humaines-et-sociales/accompagner-parents-d-enfants-tyranniques-programme-en-13-seances-0

Garcia, A. M., Sapyta, J. J., Moore, P. S. et al. (2010). Predictors and moderators of treatment outcome in the Pediatric Obsessive Compulsive Treatment Study. *Journal of the American Academy of Child and Adolescent Psychiatry*, *49*, 1024–1033. https://doi.org/10.1016/j.jaac.2010.06.013 PMID:20855047

Goddard, N., Van Gink, K., Van der Stegen, B., Van Driel, J., & Cohen, A. P. (2009). "Smeed het ijzer als het koud is." Non-Violent Resistance op een acuut psychiatrische afdeling voor adolescenten. *Maandblad Geestelijke Volksgezondheid*, *64*, 531–539.

Golan, O., Shilo, H., & Omer, H. (2018). Non-violent resistance parent training for the parents of young adults with High Functioning Autism Spectrum Disorder. *Journal of Family Therapy*, *40*, 4–24. https://onlinelibrary.wiley.com/doi/abs/10.1111/1467-6427.12106

Gold, L. H., & Frierson, R. L. (eds.) (2020). *Textbook of suicide risk assessment and management*. American Psychiatric Association Publishing.

Haley, J. (1980). *Leaving home*. McGraw Hill.

Harvey, L. J., Hunt, C., & White, F. A. (2019). Dialectical Behavior Therapy for emotion regulation difficulties: A systematic review. *Behaviour Change*, *36*, 143–164. https://doi.org/10.1017/bec.2019.9

Hooven, C. (2013). Parents-CARE: A suicide prevention program for parents of at-risk youth. *Journal of Child and Adolescent Psychiatric Nursing*, *26*, 85–95. https://doi.org/10.1111/jcap.12025 PMID:23351111

Jakob, P. (2019). Child focussed family therapy using non-violent resistance. Hearing the voice of need in the traumatised child. In E. Heismann, J. Jude & E. Day (eds.), *Non-violent resistance innovations in practice* (pp. 51–63). Pavillion.

Johnson, J. G., Cohen, P., Gould, M. S. et al. (2002). Childhood adversities, interpersonal difficulties, and risk for suicide attempts during late adolescence and early adulthood. *Archives of General Psychiatry*, *59*(8), 741–749. https://doi.org/10.1001/archpsyc.59.8.741 PMID:12150651

Kashani, J. H., Goddard, P., & Reid, J. C. (1989). Correlates of suicidal ideation in a community sample of children and adolescents. *Journal of the American Academy of Child and Adolescent Psychiatry, 28*(6), 912–917. https://jaacap.org/article/S0890-8567(09)60216-1/pdf PMID: 2808262

King, C. A., Arango, A., Kramer, A. et al. (2019). Association of the Youth-Nominated Support Team Intervention for Suicidal Adolescents with 11- to 14-Year Mortality Outcomes: Secondary Analysis of a Randomized Clinical Trial. *JAMA Psychiatry, 76* (5), 492–498. https://jamanetwork.com/article.aspx?doi=10.1001/jamapsychiatry.2018.4358 PMID:30725077

Lavi-Levavi, I., Shachar, I., & Omer, H. (2013). Training in non-violent resistance for parents of violent children: Differences between fathers and mothers. *Journal of Systemic Therapies, 32*, 79–93. https://doi.org/10.1521/jsyt.2013.32.4.79

Lebowitz, E., & Omer, H. (2013). *Treating child and adolescent anxiety: A guide for caregivers.* Wiley and Sons. https://doi.org/10.1002/9781118589366

Lebowitz, E., Dolberger, D., Nortov, E., & Omer, H. (2012). Parent training in nonviolent resistance for adult entitled dependence. *Family Process, 51*, 90–106. https://onlinelibrary.wiley.com/doi/abs/10.1111/j.1545-5300.2012.01382.x PMID:22428713

Lebowitz, E., Omer, H., Hermes, H., & Scahill, L. (2014). Parent Training for Childhood Anxiety Disorders: The SPACE Program. *Cognitive and Behavioral Practice, 21*(4), 456–469. https://doi.org/10.1016/j.cbpra.2013.10.004

Lebowitz, E. R., Marin, C., Martino, A., Shimshoni, Y., & Silverman, W. K. (2020). Parent-Based Treatment as Efficacious as Cognitive-Behavioral Therapy for Childhood Anxiety: A Randomized Noninferiority Study of Supportive Parenting for Anxious Childhood Emotions. *Journal of the American Academy of Child and Adolescent Psychiatry, 59*(3), 362–372. https://doi.org/10.1016/j.jaac.2019.02.014 PMID:30851397

Li, T. M., & Wong, P. W. (2015). Youth social withdrawal behavior (hikikomori): A systematic review of qualitative and quantitative studies. *The Australian and New Zealand Journal of Psychiatry, 49*(7), 595–609. https://doi.org/10.1177/00048 67415581179 PMID:25861794

Lothringer-Sagi, Z. (2020). Vigilant care among juvenile offenders: Development of a short-term intervention and an analysis of its efficiency and theoretical basis. Doctoral dissertation, Tel Aviv University, Tel Aviv.

Miller, A. L., Rathus, J. H., & Linehan, M. M. (2017). *Dialectical Behavior Therapy with suicidal adolescents.* Guilford Press.

OECD. (2016). The NEET challenge: What can be done for jobless and disengaged youth? In *Society at a glance 2016: OECD social indicators.* OECD Publishing. https://doi.org/10.1787/9789264261488-en

OECD. (2019). Youth not in employment, education or training (NEET) (indicator). doi:10.1787/72d1033a-en

Omer, H. (1999). *Parental presence: Reclaiming a leadership role in bringing up our children.* Zeig, Tucker & Teisen.

Omer, H. (2004a). Helping parents deal with children's acute disciplinary problems without escalation: The principle of nonviolent resistance. *Family Process, 40*(1), 53–66. https://onlinelibrary.wiley.com/doi/abs/10.1111/j.1545-5300.2001.40101000 53.x PMID:11288370

Omer, H. (2004b). *Nonviolent resistance. A new approach to violent and self-destructive children.* Cambridge University Press.

Omer, H. (2011). *The new authority: Family, school and community*. Cambridge University Press.

Omer, H. (2017). *Parental vigilant care. A guide for clinicians and caretakers*. Routledge. https://doi.org/10.4324/9781315624976

Omer, H. (in press). *Non-violent resistance: A new approach for violent and self-destructive children (new edition)*. Cambridge University Press.

Omer, H., & Dolberger, D. I. (2015). Helping parents cope with suicide threats: An approach based on nonviolent resistance. *Family Process, 54*, 559–575. https://doi.org/10.1111/famp.12129 PMID:25594236

Omer, H., & Lebowitz, E. R. (2016). Nonviolent resistance. Helping caregivers reduce problematic behaviors in children and adolescents. *Journal of Marital and Family Therapy, 42*(4), 688–700. https://doi.org/10.1111/jmft.12168 PMID:27292182

Omer, H., Schorr-Sapir, I., & Efron, R. (2016). Behandlungsprotokoll fuer Schullverweigerung. In C. A. Rexroth & T. Lustig (eds.), *Schulvermeidung* (pp. 33–58). Vandenhoeck & Ruprecht. https://doi.org/10.14220/9783737005616.33

Omer, H., Steinmetz, S. G., Carthy, T., & von Schlippe, A. (2013). The anchoring function: Parental authority and the parent-child bond. *Family Process, 52*(2), 193–206. https://doi.org/10.1111/famp.12019 PMID:23763680

Pozza, A., Coluccia, A., Kato, T., Gaetani, M., & Ferretti, F. (2019). The 'Hikikomori' syndrome: Worldwide prevalence and co-occurring major psychiatric disorders: A systematic review and meta-analysis protocol. *BMJ Open, 9*, e025213. https://bmjopen.bmj.com/content/9/9/e025213 PMID:31542731

Rothmann-Kabir, Y. (2018). Applying "The New Authority" model in families of poorly balanced adolescents with type 1 diabetes. Doctoral dissertation, Tel Aviv University, Tel Aviv. https://tau-primo.hosted.exlibrisgroup.com/permalink/f/bqa2g2/972TAU_ALMA51310479870004146

Schorr-Sapir, I. (2018). *The efficacy of "nonviolent resistance" parent training for treating ADHD in children*. Tel-Aviv University.

Sela, Y. (2019). Examining efficacy of "technological parental monitoring" versus "parental vigilant care" for reducing problematic internet usage among adolescents. Doctoral dissertation, Tel Aviv University, Tel Aviv.

Sharp, G. (1973). *The politics of nonviolent action*. Extending Horizons Books.

Shimshoni, Y., & Lebowitz, E. R. (2020). Childhood avoidant/restrictive food intake disorder: Review of treatments and a novel parent-based approach. *Journal of Cognitive Psychotherapy. 1;34*(3), 200–224. doi:10.1891/JCPSY-D-20-00009 PMID: 32817402

Shimshoni, Y., Farah, H., Lotan, T. et al. (2015). Effects of parental vigilant care and feedback on novice driver risk. *Journal of Adolescence, 38*, 69–80. https://doi.org/10.1016/j.adolescence.2014.11.002 PMID:25480357

Shimshoni, Y., Shrinivasa, B., Cherian, A. V., & Lebowitz, E. R. (2019). Family accommodation in psychopathology: A synthesized review. *Indian Journal of Psychiatry, 61*(Suppl 1), S93–S103. https://doi.org/10.4103/psychiatry.IndianJPsychiatry_530_18 PMID:30745682

Shneidman, E. S. (1985). *Definition of suicide*. Jason Aronson.

Stanley, B., Brown, G., Brent, D. A. et al. (2009). Cognitive-behavioral therapy for suicide prevention (CBT-SP): Treatment model, feasibility, and acceptability. *Journal of the American Academy of Child and Adolescent Psychiatry, 48*(10), 1005–1013. https://doi.org/10.1097/CHI.0b013e3181b5dbfe PMID:19730273

Steinberg, L. (2014). The case for delayed adulthood, The New York Times. September 19, 2019. www.nytimes.com/2014/09/21/opinion/sunday/the-case-for-delayed-adulthood .html

Storch, E. A., Geffken, G. R., Merlo, L. J. et al. (2007). Family accommodation in pediatric obsessive-compulsive disorder. *Journal of Clinical Child and Adolescent Psychology*, *36*, 207–216. https://doi.org/10.1080/15374410701277929 PMID:17484693

Tajan, N. (2015). Japanese post-modern social renouncers: An exploratory study of the narratives of Hikikomori subjects. *Subjectivity*, *8*(3), 283–304. https://doi.org/10 .1057/sub.2015.11

Tamaki, S. (2013). *Hikikomori: Adolescence without end*. Trans. Jeffrey Angles. University of Minnesota Press.

Teo, A. R., & Gaw, A. C. (2010). Hikikomori, a Japanese culture-bound syndrome of social withdrawal?: A proposal for DSM-5. *The Journal of Nervous and Mental Disease*, *198*(6), 444–449. doi:10.1097/NMD.0b013e3181e086b1

Uchida, Y., & Norasakkunkit, V. (2015). The NEET and Hikikomori spectrum: Assessing the risks and consequences of becoming culturally marginalized. *Frontiers in psychology*, *6*, 1117. https://doi.org/10.3389/fpsyg.2015.01117

US Census Bureau. (2018). Historical marital status tables revised: November 14, 2018. www.census.gov/data/tables/time-series/demo/families/marital.html

Van Gink, K. (2019). Strike while the iron is cold. The adaptation, implementation and effectiveness of non-violent resistance in residential settings for children and adolescents. Doctoral dissertation, VU University, Amsterdam, the Netherlands. https://research.vu.nl /en/publications/strike-while-the-iron-is-cold-the-adaptation-implementation-and-e

Van Holen, F., Vanderfaeillie, J., & Omer, H. (2016). Adaptation and evaluation of a nonviolent resistance intervention for foster parents: A progress report. *Journal of Marital and Family Therapy*, *42*(2), 256–271. https://doi.org/10.1111/jmft.12125 PMID:25907660

Van Holen, F., Vanderfaeillie, J., Omer, H., & Vanschoonlandt, F. (2018). Training in non-violent resistance for foster parents. *Research on Social Work Practice*, *28*(8), 931–942. https://doi.org/10.1177/1049731516662915

Vespa, J. (2017). The changing economics and demographics of young adulthood: 1975–2016. U.S. Census Bureau. www.census.gov/content/dam/Census/library/pub lications/2017/demo/p20-579.pdf

Wagner, B. M., Silverman, M. A. C., & Martin, C. E. (2003). Family factors in youth suicidal behaviors. *The American Behavioral Scientist*, *46*(9), 1171–1191. https://doi .org/10.1177/0002764202250661

Wyman, P. A., Brown, C. H., Inman, J. et al. (2008). Randomized trial of a gatekeeper program for suicide prevention: 1-year impact on secondary school staff. *Journal of Consulting and Clinical Psychology*, *76*(1), 104–115. https://doi.org/10.1037/0022- 006X.76.1.104 PMID:18229988

Zalewski, M., Lewis, J. K., & Martin, C. G. (2018). Identifying novel applications of dialectical behavior therapy: Considering emotion regulation and parenting. *Current Opinion in Psychology*, *21*, 122–126. 10.1016/j.copsyc.2018.02.013 PMID:29529427

Index

accommodation, 1–2, 8
  and cohabitation, 77
  and dysfunction, 19, 24, 39, 82
  and high-functioning autistic disorder, 29
  and self-sacrifice, 24
  automatic, 57
  behaviors, 13, 55, 88, 118
  damages of, 43, 52
  difficulty of stopping, 40
  discussing during intervention, 51
  effects of, 39, 40
  justification of, 35
  NVR and reducing, 5
  services, 12
  versus support, 19
adolescence, 9, 31–32, 95, 97, 101, 103, 139
  adult-child's, 61
  extended, 7, 14, 21
  social withdrawal in, 96, 101
adolescents, 1, 16–17, 32–33, 48, 95, 96,
    101–103, 105–106, 108, 145
adolescents, and suicide threats, 85–86, 94
adolescents at risk, 95–108
adult-children, 1, 51, 70, 80
  infantilizing beliefs, 72
  life narrative, 132
  parents of, 22
  perceived incapacity, 12, 34
  reactions to de-accommodation, 74
  survival mode, 9
  use of family home, 73
adult-child's expectations, 36, 82
adulthood, 7, 11, 14, 17, 32, 96–97, 101, 139
  and notion of independence, 17
  chasm with adolescence, 14
  early, 32, 103, 143
  fails to emerge, 15
  normative, 17
  psychosocial, 11, 95
  send off to, 16
  spontaneous passage to, 16
  the journey to, 11

  transition to as crisis, 15
adults, 11, 18, 38, 39, 68, 86, 95
  born in the 1950s and 60s, 14
  parents of, 32, 95
  young, 1, 15, 93, 143
anchoring, 22, 84–85, 88
  function, 32
  phase, 84, 86
  self, 88
announcement, 8, 55, 57, 58, 59, 60, 61, 84, 91,
    100, 121
  after, 69, 87, 98
  and school avoidance, 102
  and suicide threat, 87
  as controlled crisis, 111
  clear formulation, 59
  delivering, 91
  in crisis situations, 109
  preparing, 59–60, 61
  text, 60, 65, 97
  to older parents, 113
  without having met supporters, 61
anxiety, 32, 41–42, 46
  and accommodation, 2, 6, 24, 51
  and de-accommodation, 71, 74, 79
  and invisible risk, 95
  disorders, 6, 13, 40, 73, 115
  effects on parents, 11
  escalating, 25
  following child's suicide attempt, 88
  overcoming, 74, 78, 132
  social, 103
  SPACE program, 40

crisis, 15, 26, 84, 109–111, 113
  and accommodation, 111
  as opportunity, 71
  financial, 115
  intervention-initiated, 111
  management, 109
  suicidal, 82, 86–88
  transition to adulthood, 15

de-accommodation, 1–2, 11–33, 39, 40, 41, 42,
    43, 45, 51, 52, 56–57, 65–66, 68–74,
    87–88, 111, 115–116, 135
  and fear of suicide, 45
  as third intervention stage, 49, 63
  outcomes, 52
  parents' difficulties in reducing, 40–41, 44
  risks, 47, 59
dependence, 7–8, 14, 15, 16–18
  and independence, 7, 16–17, 140
  bond, 13, 34, 48, 53, 82, 89, 116
  dysfunctional, 9, 11, 12, 47–48, 51, 61, 78,
    82, 118
  financially irresponsible, 105
  functional, 17–18
  on screens, 96
disability, 28
disorder, 13, 30, 40–41
  avoidant personality disorder, 93
  bipolar, 48
  eating, 7, 40, 48
  high-functioning autistic, 143
  obsessive compulsive, 13, 32, 39, 48, 73,
    114, 146
  oppositional-defiant, 6, 13
  personality disorder, 48, 119
  psychotic outbreak, 115
  PTSD, 48
  schizophrenia, 13, 48, 114

emerging adulthood, 7, 14–15, 140
  theory, 14–15
emerging adults, 15, 29, 142
  parents of, 16
entitled dependence
  as a trans-diagnostic condition, 14, 139
  as systemic problem, 36
  blaming rituals, 44
entitlement, 28, 105
  adult-child's, 12, 14, 29, 30, 109
entrenched dependence, 1, 7
  and clinical conditions, 13
  and "invisible risk" in adolescence,
    95
  and NEET, 139
  and social avoidance, 134
  as coconstructed reality, 47
  as relational pattern, 34
  coercive nature, 31
  from childhood to adulthood, 32
entrenched dependence, in psychiatric
    context, 114
escalation, 8–9, 44, 47, 49, 53–55, 56–57,
    69–70, 82, 88
  complementary, 44, 82, 88

  preventing, 53, 99
  symmetrical, 44, 82

family therapy, 36
fear, 9, 11–33, 41–45, 56, 61–62, 103–104, 136
finance, 11–12, 21, 28, 30, 58, 68–69, 106–108,
    110, 126
  coaching, 28, 33, 67, 68, 108, 110
  independence, 16–17
  irresponsible behavior, 9, 95, 105

Hikikomori, 145
internet, 30, 48, 60, 63, 72
  addiction, 67, 105, 114
  connectivity, 99
  shutdown, 99

interpersonal patterns, 1, 7, 12, 15, 29, 32, 34,
    53, 84
  coercive, 87, 91
  dependence–accommodation
    relationship, 139
intervention, 7, 9, 13, 46, 61–62, 109, 119
  and police involvement, 68
  and psychiatric care, 68
  and social workers, 68
  duration of, 47
  for suicide threats, 88, 142
  in emergencies, 109
  preventive, 112, 139
  process of, 69, 74, 109, 114
isolation, 6, 9, 11–33, 61, 63, 71, 82,
    85–86, 104
  adult-child's, 13
  and suicide threats, 85
  family's, 29, 61

NEET (not in education, employment or
    training), 1, 7, 11, 14, 139, 144
Non-Violent Resistance. See NVR.
not in education, employment or training. See
    NEET.
NVR
  and entrenched dependence, 10, 140
  and reducing accommodation, 6
  announcement typifies, 8
  contra-indication, 93
  goal of, 39, 82
  group therapy, 104
  importance of parental resistance, 57, 103
  in the psychiatric ward, 118
  interventions, 9–10, 32, 94
  manuals, 8
  parental, 6, 8
  practitioners, 53

program, 55, 83, 113
program for suicide threats, 83
resistance, 8–9, 32–33, 58, 69, 71, 87, 89, 98,
    100–101
sensitizes parents, 6
societies, 32
sociopolitical model, 6
therapists, 37, 92
training, 43–45, 53, 115
NVR (Non-Violent Resistance), 1, 6, 8

OECD, 1, 139

parental role, 84, 87
parental services, 48, 51, 55, 79, 88, 91, 94
    financial, 72
    reducing or withholding, 71, 77
    victimhood, 71
parents
    accommodation, 24, 28, 116
    authority, 94
    courageous, 10
    de-accommodation, 70, 71, 74
    effacement, 21
    elderly, 18, 68
    firmness, 43, 54
    guilt, 34
    isolation, 52
    objections, 43, 62
    parental home, 11, 51–52, 60–61, 66, 76–79,
        111–112, 125, 127
    protectiveness, 13, 34, 44, 51, 113, 127
    sacrifice, 8, 24–25, 26, 113
    time perspective, 7, 18, 20, 49
privacy, 28, 64, 74–75, 77, 86, 140
    reduction of rights, 71, 74, 85
    reflex, 62
    rights, 73, 74, 76–77
provocations, 49, 53, 91
psychiatry, 68
    diagnosis, 14, 48
    emergency center, 68
    inpatient, 68, 109, 115–116
    psychiatrist, 23, 33, 35, 67, 68, 92–93,
        114–115, 136, 137
    ward, 7, 9, 88, 115, 116, 117–120
psychopathology, 2, 93, 139, 145
psychotherapy, 1, 13, 24, 30, 35, 115, 119
    refusal, 19, 34, 115

rehabilitation, 28, 68, 119
    agencies, 29, 33, 67, 68, 121

school refusal, 9, 43, 95, 101–103, 105
screen addiction, 96–99, 101

secrets and secrecy, 11, 31, 41, 44, 61, 70,
    85, 86
    and shame, 43
    and social isolation, 34
    breaking taboo, 71, 74
    disclosing, 58, 60, 63, 80, 85
    fear of disclosure, 13
    versus transparency in NVR, 56
self-regulation, 140
shame, 11, 33, 43–44, 52, 62, 80, 104
social services, 76, 77, 113
suicide threats, 9, 13, 29–31, 45, 61–62, 65,
    81–89, 90–91, 92–94, 119, 142–144, 146
    and NVR, 83
    and "parliament of the mind," 84
    and secrecy, 85
    and suicide risk, 82–83
    containment and anchoring phases, 84
    effects of social support, 86
    suicide watch, 85, 86
    typical parent reactions to, 83
support
    financial, 16
    functional versus dysfunctional, 19
    gathering, 29, 52, 55, 56, 58, 59, 61–62
    network, 33, 49, 61
supporters, 8–9, 42–44, 52, 54–55, 61–64,
    65–67, 72–76, 84–87, 91–93, 98–99,
    109–111, 121
symptoms, 24, 29, 40, 93, 114
    manic, 93
    paranoid, 29
systemic, 31, 139

taboos, breaking, 74, 109
therapist, 8–9, 11–33, 37, 45–46, 49–52, 56–57,
    61–70, 77–79, 109–112, 125–126,
    132–138
    adult-child's, 57, 67
    position, 49, 51, 64–65, 111
    psychiatric help, 33
therapy, 8, 9, 19–20, 21–24, 29–33, 35–39, 46,
    56–57, 78–79, 123–124, 131–132,
    133–136, 137–138
    acceptance by the adult child, 8
    end of, 78
    first session, 26, 79
    goals, 8, 46, 49, 52, 91
    individual, 8, 9
    integrity, 8
    parent-initiated, 35
    plan, 8, 55–56
    refusal, 8, 35
    stages, 8
    therapeutic alliance, 8, 45, 62, 109, 112

therapy (cont.)
  therapeutic plowing, 51
  therapeutic system, 68
  without the adult child's involvement, 36
threats, 11–33, 45, 65–66, 81–85, 87,
    100, 127
total responsibility
  assumption of, 8, 52
  sense of, 39, 61
total responsibility narrative, 38–39, 47, 52, 62,
    68, 72, 141

traditional psychotherapy's, 140
training in Non-Violent Resistance, 40,
    144, 146
treatment (see therapy)

violence, 8–9, 20, 31–32, 46, 61–62, 65–68, 71,
    76, 78–79, 83, 105, 115
  children, 144
  chronic, 140
  domestic, 74
  verbal, 105

For EU product safety concerns, contact us at Calle de José Abascal, 56–1°,
28003 Madrid, Spain or eugpsr@cambridge.org.

www.ingramcontent.com/pod-product-compliance
Ingram Content Group UK Ltd.
Pitfield, Milton Keynes, MK11 3LW, UK
UKHW010251140625
459647UK00013BA/1786